D0240594

RUDE
Health

Published in 2012 by Prion

an imprint of the Carlton Publishing Group
20 Mortimer Street
London W1T 3JW

10 9 8 7 6 5 4 3 2 1

Copyright © 2012 Carlton Books Limited

All rights reserved. This book is sold subject to the
condition that it shall not, by way of trade or otherwise, be
lent, resold, hired out or otherwise circulated without the
publisher's prior written consent in any form of cover or
binding other than that which it is published and without a
similar condition, including this condition, being imposed
upon the subsequent purchaser.

ISBN 978-1-85375-878-2

A CIP catalogue record of this book can be obtained from
the British Library.

Printed and bound in Great Britain by CPI Group (UK) Ltd,
Croydon CR0 4YY

RUDE
Health

A healthy dose of stories and one-liners

that will have you in stitches!

Introduction

There's really nothing funny about sickness, accidents, mental disorders or geriatrics... but, for some reason, the medical profession has always provided a rich vein of humour.

I mean, hospitals? They're terrible places. Smelly, uncomfortable, full of ill people. If that sounds like a place you'd like to visit, there must be something wrong with you...

Here's a book packed full of seizure-inducing medical mirth, one-liners and sick gags. There are jokes about homeopathy, Viagra, NHS Direct, STDs, chiropractors, nutritionists, hospital food, randy nurses and plenty of "Doctor, Doctor" gags.

Administer to your funny bone as required.

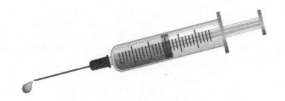

Contents

At the Doctor's

I went to see the doctor yesterday.
"What seems to be the problem, George?"
he asked.
"Well, I think I suffer from schizophrenia,"
I said, being Frank.

An elderly couple go to their doctor for a check up. The man goes in first. "How're you doing?" asks the doctor. "Pretty good," answers the old man. "I'm eating well, and I'm still in control of my bowels and bladder. In fact, when I get up at night to pee, the good Lord turns the light on for me."

The doctor decides not to comment on that last statement, and goes into the next room to check on the man's wife. "How're you feeling?" he asks.

"I'm doing well," answers the old woman. "I still have lots of energy and I'm not feeling any pain."

The doctor says, "That's nice. It sounds like you and your husband are both doing well."

"One thing though – your husband said that when he gets up to pee at night, the good Lord turns the light on for him. Do you have any idea what he means?"

"Oh no," says the woman, "he's peeing in the refrigerator again."

"Doctor, doctor, my wooden leg is giving me a lot of pain."

"Why's that?"

"My wife keeps hitting me over the head with it."

8

A man walks sheepishly into the doctor's office. The doctor asks him what's wrong and the man sighs and pulls down his trousers to reveal a penis full of holes.

"It's terrible!" says the man. "It's like a garden sprinkler. Every time I go to the loo, I piss all over my shoes!"

The doc looks at it for a while, and then scribbles a note. "I'm going to have to refer you to Mr Venables."

"Why?" asks the man. "Is he a specialist?"

"No," replies the doctor, "he's a clarinet player – he'll show you how to hold it properly."

Doctor: I have some good news and some bad news, which would you like to hear first?

Patient: Uhhh, well, give me the bad news first, I guess.

Doctor: You only have one week left to live.

Patient: Oh no! What good news can you possibly tell me now?

Doctor: Well, you know that really hot-looking nurse who just came in here? I'm taking her out to dinner tonight, and who knows what could happen!

> *A man went to the doctor.*
> *The doctor examined him and said: "I'm sorry to have to tell you this – but you only have three minutes left to live."*
> *The man said: "Oh my god! Are you sure there is nothing you can do for me?"*
> *The doctor thought for a moment then replied: "I could boil you an egg!"*

An elderly lady is being attended to by her doctor. A few minutes into the examination, a screeching comes from the room, and then the lady bursts out of the room as quick as she can possibly move.

The receptionist intercepts her, calms her down and eventually manages to discover the problem. Angrily, the receptionist barges into the doctor's office and screams, "Shame on you, Mrs. Jones is 82 years old, and you told her she's pregnant!"

The doctor continues writing calmly and barely looking up says, "Ahh, yes. But, does she still have the hiccups?"

> *A man goes to see the doctor and says, "Doctor, I have this awful empty feeling, I'm as listless as a Welsh resort in winter." The doctor replies, "Oh dear, it sounds like you're Rhyl."*

"Doctor, doctor, I can't keep my hands from shaking."

"Do you drink a lot?"

"No, I spill most of it."

Doctor: Have you ever had this before?
Patient: Yes.
Doctor: Well, you've got it again.

A man goes to see his GP in a real panic. "You've got to help me Doc," he plead. "I can't stop shoplifting. One of these days I'm going to get caught and I'll end up behind bars with my life ruined."

"Lucky you came in today," replies the doctor. "We've got these brand new pills in. Take two every morning – hopefully that'll solve the problem."

"But what if they don't work – what am I going to do?"

"Well if they don't cure you... see if you can get me an iPad."

"Doctor, doctor, I keep being told I'm a wheelbarrow."

"You mustn't let people push you around."

A man with a glass eye had been out for a night on the town. Being the worse for wear, when he stumbled into bed, he dropped his glass eye into his drinking water on the bed table. During the night, he drank the water and swallowed the eye.

A day or so later he was suffering from severe constipation, so he went to his local surgery. The doctor inserted his proctoscope and muttered under his breath, "Good grief, I've looked up plenty of backsides before, but this is the first one to ever look back at me."

Patient: Doctor, I think I swallowed a pillow.
Doctor: How do you feel?
Patient: A little down in the mouth.

A man walked into a doctor's office.

What do you have?" the receptionist asked him.

"Shingles," he replied.

She told him to sit down.

Soon a nurse called him and asked, "What do you have?"

"Shingles," he replied.

She took his blood pressure, weight, and complete medical history. Then she took him to a room, told him to remove all of his clothes, and left.

After a few minutes the doctor came in and asked, "What do you have?"

"Shingles," the man told him.

The doctor looked him up and down and asked, "Where? I don't see them."

"Out on the truck. Where do you want me to unload them?"

A doctor remarked on his patient's rather ruddy complexion. "I know," the patient said. "It's high blood pressure, it's from my family.

"Your mother's side or father's side?" questioned the doctor. "Neither, it's from my wife's side. "What?" the doctor said, "that can't be true. You can't get high blood pressure from your wife's family."

"Oh yeah?" the patient responded, "you should meet them sometime!"

Mother: I need to speak to the doctor, it's an emergency – my child has a temperature of 101.

Doctor (to Receptionist): Find out how she's taking the temperature.

Receptionist: How are you taking it?

Mother: Oh, I'm holding up OK so far.

A woman accompanied her husband to the doctor's office. After his check-up, the doctor asked for the wife to come into his office for a private word.

He told her, "Your husband is suffering from a very severe disease, combined with horrible stress. If you don't do the following, your husband will surely die."

"Each morning, fix him a healthy breakfast. Be pleasant, and make sure he is in a good mood. For lunch make him a nutritious meal. For dinner prepare an especially nice meal for him. Don't burden him with chores, as he probably had a hard day. Don't discuss your problems with him; it will only make his stress worse. And most importantly, you should satisfy his every whim sexually several times a week.

"If you can do this for the next 10 months to a year, I think your husband will regain his health completely."

On the way home, the husband asked his wife, "What did the doctor say?"

"You're going to die," she replied.

A mother complained to her doctor about her daughter's strange eating habits.

"All day long she lies in bed and eats yeast and car wax," she moaned. I'm really concerned about the long term effects of her lifestyle. What will happen to her, doc?"

"Don't worry" said the Doctor, "eventually she will rise and shine!"

"Doctor, doctor, you've got to help me. Every night I dream I wrote The Lord of the Rings."

"Don't worry; you've just been Tolkien in your sleep."

"Doctor, doctor, I keep seeing images of Mickey Mouse and Donald Duck!"

"I see, and how long have you been having these Disney spells?"

"Doctor, doctor, I keep thinking I'm a pocket watch."

"Relax, you're just a bit wound up."

"Doctor, doctor, I keep thinking I'm a bucket."

"Hmmm... you do look a little pail."

"Doctor, doctor, How can I avoid catching McGilligan's disease?"

"Stay away from McGilligan."

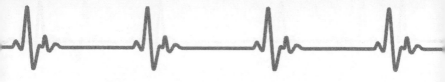

A man walked into the office of the eminent psychiatrist
Dr. Feldberg, and sat down to explain his complaint.
"Doctor, doctor! I've got this problem," the man said. "I keep
hallucinating that I'm a dog. It's crazy. I don't know what to do."
"Ahh. You are suffering from a common canine complex,"
said the doctor soothingly. "Relax. Come here and lie down on
the couch."
"Oh no, Doctor," the man said nervously, "I'm not allowed up on
the furniture."

A blonde with two red ears went to her doctor. The doctor
asked her what had happened to her ears.
"I was ironing a shirt and the phone rang – but instead of
picking up the phone I accidentally picked up the iron and
stuck it to my ear."
"Oh dear!" the doctor exclaimed in disbelief. "But... what
happened to your other ear?"
"The son-of-a-bitch called back."

"Doctor, doctor, I can't pronounce my Fs, Ts
or Hs."

"Well you can't say 'fairer than that'."

A woman went to her doctor for a follow up visit after the doctor
had prescribed testosterone (a male hormone) for her. She was a
little worried about some of the side effects she was experiencing.
Doctor: Did you take my advice of drinking a glass of cold milk
after a hot bath?
Patient: I tried but I've still got a bucket of bathwater to get
through.

15

"Doctor, doctor, there's a strawberry growing out the top of my head."

"I'll give you some cream to put on that."

"Doctor, doctor will this ointment you've given me clear up my spots?"

"You know me, I never make rash promises!"

"Doctor, doctor, – It's so annoying – I keep saying 'Aaa, Eee, I, oooh! You' at really inappropriate times."

"I think you may have irritable vowel syndrome."

"Doctor, doctor, – I keep comparing things with something else."

"Don't worry, it's only analogy"

At the Chemist

A woman goes into a chemist. "Excuse me," she asks. "Do you have any Sudocreme please?" "Ah yes Madam," replies the pharmacist. "Please, walk this way."
"If I could walk that way I wouldn't need the cream."

A woman went to a chemist to collect some Viagra tablets for her husband. "Tell him to swallow them quickly," the pharmacist advised. "Or he could get a stiff neck."

A woman asked the pharmacist if he had anything for hiccups. Quick as you like, the chemist slapped her around the face. "I bet that's stopped your hiccups," he said proudly. "No," replied the woman. "My sister waiting in the car has them."

After receiving his medication from the pharmacist, the customer asks, "Are these time release pills?"
The pharmacist replies, "Yes. They begin to work after your cheque clears."

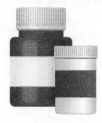

A fellow with a bad cough comes in to the chemist's, walks up to the counter and asks for the pharmacist. A young assistant tells him that the pharmacist is not available. So the man asks the assistant if he can recommend anything for his cough.

The assistant gives him a bottle of some medicine for his cough. The customer takes a big swig, then after a few minutes, with no apparent relief, he takes another, and another.

In a short while, the pharmacist returns, and sees his old friend, the customer with the cough, sitting on a bench outside. He remarks to his assistant that the fellow has never stopped at the bench before.

The assistant proudly tells the pharmacist the story of his transaction. The pharmacist looks at the recommended medication and angrily reprimands the assistant for recommending a laxative, instead of cough syrup.

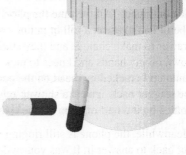

The clerk looks out at the man and comments "Well, it seems to have done the job, he's not coughing any more. The pharmacist replies, "Of course not you idiot, now he's afraid to cough!"

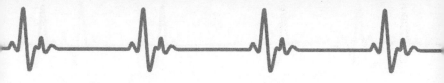

Upon arriving home, a husband was met at the door by his sobbing wife.

Tearfully she explained, "It's the pharmacist – he insulted me terribly this morning on the phone." Immediately the husband drove into town to confront the chemist and demand an apology.

Before he could say more than a word or two, the pharmacist had interrupted: "Now just a minute – listen to my side of it. This morning the alarm failed to go off, so I was late getting up. I went without breakfast and hurried out to the car, just to realize that I'd locked the house with both house and car keys inside. I had to break a window to get my keys. Then, driving a little too fast, I got a speeding ticket. Later, when I was about a mile from the shop, I had a flat tyre. When I finally got to the shop there was a bunch of people waiting for me to open up. I eventually got the shop opened, ignored the ringing phone and started to serve the queue."

He continued, "All the time the phone was ringing off the hook. Then I had to break a roll of pound coins against the cash register drawer to make change, and they spilled all over the floor. I got down on my hands and knees to pick up the coins and when I came up I cracked my head on the open cash drawer, which made me stagger back against a showcase with a bunch of perfume bottles on it... half of them hit the floor and broke.

Meanwhile, the phone is still ringing with no let up, and I finally got back to answer it. It was your wife – she wanted to know how to use a rectal thermometer – and believe me, Sir, I told her!

My mum takes so many Iron tablets the only time she feels good is when she's facing magnetic north. My brothers are fighting over her mineral rights.

A young girl asked her friend,
"What is that you're taking – the pill?"

"No it's a valium. I forgot to take the pill."

The definition of a 'miracle' drug: Anything that will do 25% as much as the label says.

Have you heard about the pharmaceutical company that developed a new drug which, when administered to women, compels them to go join a convent? The government refused to license it, though. Seems it was habit-forming.

A duck goes into a chemist's and asks for some lip balm. "Certainly sir," says the assistant, "will you be paying for this by cash or by card?" "Just put it on my bill," says the duck.

A man rings his local chemist:
"Do you sell incontinence pants?"
"Yes, sir," replies the chemist,"can I ask you where you're ringing from?"
The man replies, "From the waist down."

A man walks into a chemist's and asks for an anal deodorant. The chemist explains that they don't stock them. The man insists that he bought his last one from this store. The chemist asks the man to bring in his last purchase and he will try to match the product. The next day the man returns and shows the deodorant to the chemist. The words on the label read, 'To use, push up bottom.'

A small boy goes to a chemist's to buy some stomach medicine.
"Antibilious?" asks the chemist.
'No," replies the boy. "They're for my uncle."

> *A man walks into a chemist's and says,*
> *"I would like to buy some deodorant please."*
> *"Certainly, sir," says the chemist,*
> *"ball or aerosol?"*
> *"Neither,' says the man. "It's for my armpits."*

A man went into a chemist's shop and said, "Have you got anything for laryngitis?"
The chemist said "Good morning sir. What can I do for you?"

The doctor has prescribed me anti-hypochondria tablets. I'm not stupid I know they are only placebos – but I can't help worrying about the possible side effects.

A man went for an interview for a job as a TV news broadcaster. The interview went quite well but the trouble was he kept winking and stammering.

The interviewer said,

"Although you have a lot of the qualities we're looking for, the fact that you keep winking and stammering disqualifies you."

"Oh, that's no problem," said the man. "If I take a couple of aspirin I stop winking and stammering for an hour."

"Show me," said the interviewer.

So the man reached into his pocket. Embarrassingly he pulled out loads of condoms of every variety – ribbed, flavoured, coloured and everything, before he found the packet of aspirin. He took the aspirin and soon talked perfectly and stopped winking.

The interviewer said,

"That's amazing, but I don't think we could employ someone who'd be womanizing all over the country."

"Excuse me!" exclaimed the man, "I'm a happily married man, not a womanizer!"

"Well how do you explain all the condoms, then?" asked the interviewer.

The man replied, "Have you ever gone into a pharmacy, stammering and winking, and asked for a packet of aspirin?"

Did you hear about the new 'morning after' pill for men? It changes their blood type.

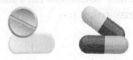

At the Hospital

A man is wheeling himself frantically down the hall of the hospital, just before his operation. An orderly stops him and asks, "What's the matter, why are you running away from the operating theatre?"

Through his gasps he replies, "Well I heard the nurse say, 'An appendectomy is a very simple operation, don't worry, I'm sure it will be all right.'"

"She was just trying to comfort you." says the orderly.

"But she wasn't talking to me; she was talking to the doctor!"

Who's the coolest doctor in the hospital?
The ultra-sound guy.
Who fills in for him when he's on holiday?
The hip-replacement guy.

Definition of Anaesthesia:
The half-awake monitoring the half-asleep while they are being half-murdered by the half-witted.

A hospital posted a notice in the nurses' rest room that said: "Remember, the first five minutes of a human being's life are the most dangerous." Underneath, a nurse had written: "The last five are pretty risky, too."

A man returns from the Middle East and is feeling very ill. He goes to see his doctor, and is immediately rushed to the hospital to undergo some tests.

The man wakes up after the tests in a private room at the hospital, and the phone by his bed rings. "This is your doctor. We have the results back from your tests and we have found you have an extremely nasty STD called G.A.S.H. It's a combination of Gonorrhoea, AIDS, Syphilis, and Herpes!"

"Oh my gosh," cried the man, "what are you going to do, doctor?"

"Well we're going to put you on a diet of pizzas, pancakes, and pitta bread," replied the doctor.

"Will that cure me?" asked the man.

The doctor replied, "Well no, but it's the only food we can slide under the door."

A woman calling her local hospital said, "Hello, I'd like to know how a patient in the East Wing is getting on."

The voice on the other end of the line said,
"What is the patient's name and room number?"

She said, "It's Beth Smith in Room E402."

He put her on hold until eventually a nurse came on:
"Oh, yes. Mrs Smith is doing very well. She's had two full meals, her blood pressure is fine, she's going to be taken off the heart monitor in a couple of hours and if she continues this improvement, Dr Nowak is going to send her home on Tuesday."

The woman said, "Thank you. That's wonderful news!"

The nurse replied, "I take it you must be a close family member or a very close friend?"

She said, "Oh no – I'm Beth Smith from E402. No one tells me a thing around here!"

A man is admitted into casualty with concussion, multiple bruises, two black eyes and a five iron wrapped tightly around his throat. The doctor asks him what happened.

"Well, it was like this," says the man, "I was having a quiet round of golf with my wife, when at the eighth hole we both sliced our balls into a field of cows. We went to look for them, and while I was rooting around, I noticed one of the cows had something white at its rear end. I walked over and lifted up the tail, and sure enough, there was a golf ball with my wife's monogram on it – stuck right in the middle of the cow's butt, that's when I made my big mistake."

"What did you do?" asks the doctor.

"Well, I lifted the cow's tail again and yelled to my wife, 'Hey, this looks like yours!' I don't remember much after that!"

A patient went into surgery to have his gall stones removed by one of the hospital's most accomplished and arrogant surgeons. The whole operation was observed by medical students. The next morning the patient woke to find his stomach perfectly stitched but with bandages around his privates.

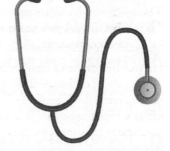

"What on earth has happened?" asked the astonished patient. No one could answer. Then one of the students came by. "Ah, it's you," he said, "well, the surgeon did such a brilliant operation that we gave him a round of applause. We clapped and clapped and clapped... so, for an encore, he circumcised you."

"I have some good news and some bad news," said the doctor, uttering a well-worn phrase.

"I'm familiar with the format," replied the patient. "First you give me the bad news."

"Oh well, that would be that I've had to amputate both your legs."

And now the bit where you give me some news that puts that dreadful event into some comic perspective?

At which point the doc goes on to say: "The man in the next bed wants to buy your slippers."

Doctor: You're coughing more easily this morning.
Patient: I should be, I've been practising all night.

Q: What is the difference between a rotweiler and a junior intensive care doctor?
A: A rotweiler lets go when you're dead!

Q: What did the patient say to the annoying doctor during liposuction surgery?
A: "Doc, you're really starting to get under my skin!"

Q. How do you hide a £5 note from a General Surgeon?
A. Hide it in the Patient's Notes.

Q. How do you hide a £5 note from an Orthopaedic Surgeon?
A. Hide it in a textbook.

Q. How do you hide a £5 note from a Plastic Surgeon?
A. Trick question – you can't.

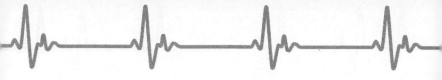

10 Things You Don't Want to Hear During Surgery

🚑 Keep hold of that, we'll need it for the autopsy.

🚑 Don't step in it. Someone call an orderly and tell them to bring a big mop.

🚑 Hey! Come back with that! Naughty dog! Bad dog!

🚑 Wait a minute, if this is his liver, then what's that?

🚑 Hand me that...uh...that uh.....long silver thingy.

🚑 Oops! Has anyone ever survived 500ml of this stuff before?

🚑 Help me out here – I'm getting one of my dizzy spells...

🚑 Everybody stand back! I lost my contact lens!

🚑 What's this doing here?

🚑 Of course it's ethical!

Just relax, the hospital staff kept telling Jim, but it was to no avail. Jim's wife was in labour and he was a nervous wreck – pacing back and forth, smoking like a chimney and biting his nails to the quick. After what seemed like a week, to both Jim and the hospital staff, a nurse came out with the happy news. "It's a girl", she cried. "Thank God, a girl!" said Jim. "At least she won't have to go suffer what I just went through!"

A young doctor just out of medical school announced to his wife that he planned to specialize in gastroenterology. When she asked him why he chose that particular field, he simply said, "There are lots of openings."

An accident-prone young surgeon is given one last chance by his bosses. His next operation is a delicate affair and all is going well until he makes an unfortunate slip and accidentally cuts off his patient's testicles. Terrified of being caught, he decides to cover-up his mistake as quickly as possible.

He inserts two onions where the testicles should be and sews the patient back up.

A month later, the man goes back for a check-up.

"Ah, I remember you," says the surgeon nervously. "Everything fine down there?"

"Well I do have a few problems and I wondered if they were common," explains the man.

"It was a pretty straightforward operation," the surgeon lies. "Tell me. What after-effects are you suffering?"

"Well Doc it's like this. I cry when I pee, my wife gets heartburn after sex and I get a hard-on when I see a cheese sandwich!"

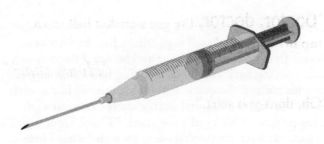

A woman's husband had been slipping in and out of a coma for several months, yet she had stayed by his bedside every single day.

One day when he came to, he motioned for her to come nearer. As she sat by him, he whispered, eyes full of tears: "You know what? You have been with me all through the bad times. When I got fired, you were there to support me. When my business failed, you were there. When I got shot, you were by my side. When we lost the house, you stayed right here. When my health started failing, you were still by my side... You know what, darling?"

"What dear?" she gently asked, smiling as her heart began to fill with warmth.

"I'm beginning to think you're f**king bad luck..."

Q: What is the difference between God and an orthopaedic surgeon?

A: God doesn't think he is an orthopaedic surgeon.

Doctor: "I have some good news and bad news for you."
Patient: "There's good news?"
Doctor: "Yes. You're going to have a disease named after you!"

"Doctor, doctor, I've got a cricket ball stuck up my backside."

"How's that?"

"Oh, don't you start."

The patient awakened after the operation to find herself in a room with all the blinds drawn.

"Why are all the blinds closed?" she asked her doctor.

"Well," the surgeon responded, "They're fighting a huge fire across the street, and we didn't want you to wake up and think the operation had failed."

Patients were often referred to physiotherapy with vague knee pain. Their diagnosis read "IDK". They were told it meant Internal Derangement of the Knee, but the nurses all knew what it really meant: "I Don't Know!"

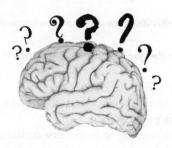

A group of children were on a school trip around a hospital. They found the room with the x-ray machines the most fascinating and were interested in finding out how they worked. The radiologist began by asked them if they had ever broken a bone? One little boy raised his hand, "Oh yeah, I did!" "Did it hurt?" She asked. "No!" replied the little lad. "Wow, you must be a very brave boy! Which bone did you break?" she enquired. As bold as brass he answered: "My sister's arm!"

Famous last words before entering A&E...

🚑   What does this button do?

🚑   It's probably just a rash.

🚑   Are you sure the power is off?

🚑   The odds of that happening have to be a million to one!

🚑   Which wire was I supposed to cut?

🚑   I wonder where the mother bear is.

🚑   I've seen this done on TV.

🚑   These are the good kind of mushrooms.

🚑   It's strong enough to take the both of us.

🚑   This doesn't taste quite right.

🚑   I can do that with my eyes closed.

🚑   Well, we've made it this far.

🚑   You wouldn't hit a guy with glasses on, would you?

🚑   Oh, don't be so superstitious!

🚑   Now watch this!

Laughter's the Best Medicine
(has no one here heard of penicillin?)

David Cameron was on the election trail visiting an old people's home. He approached one old lady and very gently asked:
"Hello my dear. What's your name?"
"Oh hello young man," she replied. She thought for a moment and said, "Ethel, yes that's it, Ethel."
And then she turned to walk away.
The Prime Minister, however, was not to be discouraged.
"And how are you Ethel?"
"I'm fine thank you," she says, now getting a bit irritated.
"Do you know who I am?" he asked.
"No." came the curt reply. "But if you ask one of the nurses, they will tell you."

A machine operator comes home from the factory and tells his wife: "Honey, I've got good news and bad news. First, the good news: I got £25,000 severance pay!"
His wife replies: "£25,000 in severance pay? That's great! Now, what's the bad news?"
"Well," he says, "wait till you hear what was severed!"

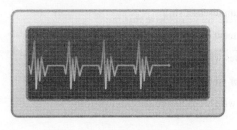

An army major is visiting sick soldiers. He goes up to one patient and asks:

"What's your problem, private?"

"Chronic syphilis, sir."

"What treatment are you getting?"

"Five minutes with the wire brush each day, sir."

"What's your ambition soldier?"

"To get back to the front, sir."

"Good man." says the Major. He goes to the next patient. "What's your problem, private?"

"Chronic piles, sir."

"What treatment are you getting?"

"Five minutes with the wire brush each day, sir."

"What's your ambition, man?"

"To get back to the front, sir."

"That's the spirit." says the Major. He goes to the next bed. "What's your problem, private?"

"Chronic gum disease, sir."

"What treatment are you getting?"

"Five minutes with the wire brush each day, sir."

"What's your ambition?"

"To get the wire brush before the other two, sir."

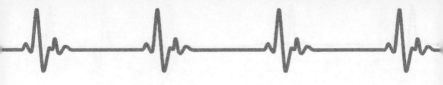

From the newspapers...

Doctors are beginning to accept that stomach ulcers are infectious. They are caused by a bug called Helicopter...

Your chance of catching an STD during your period is greater, because the blood changes the PhD level in the vagina...

Dinosaur extinction may well have occurred when a steroid hit the Earth...

He recovered from a tuna of the kidney...

Transplant surgeon has called for a ban on kidneys-for-ale operations...

In America, you can buy melatonin as a vitamin supplement. It is a hormone that your penile gland secretes when it gets dark...

We don't know why, but it seems men don't get bacterial vaginosis...

FOR SALE: Real bone half-skeleton, in better condition than seller. £250...

Lung cancer in women mushrooms...

New study of obesity looks for larger test group...

New vaccine may contain rabies...

Hospitals are sued by seven foot doctors...

Kicking baby considered to be healthy...

Never withhold herpes from loved one...

Smoking organ causes stir at nursing home...

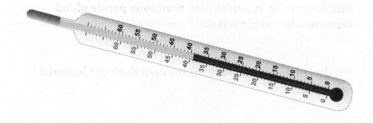

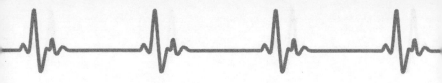

Jeff and Judy had been married three years but already their life together seemed far from perfect so they decided to attend a marriage counsellor. They sat down in his office and the therapist began work immediately.

"So who wants to begin?" he asked. "Either of you two prepared to say what they think has gone wrong?"

Judy looked up nervously and nodded. "He's so often late home from work. Sometimes he's out drinking with mates or he's wining and dining business acquaintances and sometimes I've no idea where he is."

Jeff went to interrupt, but the counsellor raised a finger to halt him as Judy was getting into full flow.

"And he never does anything to help around the house – I've have to do all the cooking and cleaning. When he's in he just sits in front of the TV."

Again Jeff opens his mouth to defend himself but is once again hushed.

"And he's never around at weekends – he's off fishing or to the football or down the pub." At this point Judy stops to wipe a tear from her eye. As she does so the counsellor walks over to her, hugs her and starts kissing her passionately. This goes on for a couple of minutes before he returns to his seat.

The couple were speechless. She sat there quite unable to believe what had happened and Jeff was open-mouthed in disbelief.

"Now," said the counsellor turning to Jeff. "She needs that and more at least twice a week." Jeff thought hard for a second before saying, "Well, I suppose I could bring her on Mondays and Wednesdays if you could fit her in."

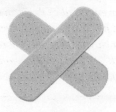

36

At Sunday school, the vicar was taking questions. A small boy put his hand up.

"Did Moses get better in the end?" he asked.

The puzzled vicar asked him why he thought he might ever have been ill.

"He must have been," replied the youngster. "Didn't God tell him to take the tablets?"

A very shy man was in the hospital for a series of tests, the last of which had left his stomach a little upset. Having already made several false-alarm trips to the bathroom, he decided the latest was another and stayed put. He suddenly filled his bed with diarrhoea and such was his embarrassment he completely lost it. In a fit of pique, he jumped up, gathered up the bed sheets, and threw them out the hospital window.

A drunk was walking by the hospital when the sheets landed on him. He started yelling, cursing, and swinging his arms wildly, which left the soiled sheets in a tangled pile at his feet. As the drunk stood there staring down at the sheets, a security guard who had watched the whole incident walked up and asked, "What the hell was that all about?" Still staring down, the drunk replied: "I think I just beat the ****out of a ghost!"

"What kind of work do you do?" a woman passenger enquired of the man travelling in her train compartment.

"I'm a Naval surgeon," he replied.

"My word!" spluttered the woman, "How you doctors specialise these days."

When a car skidded on wet pavement and struck a bollard, several bystanders ran over to help the driver. A woman was the first to reach the victim, but a man rushed in and pushed her back. "Step aside, lady," he barked. "I've just this minute taken a course in first aid." He got out his course book and began to methodically follow the instructions.

The woman continued to watch him for a minute, before tapping his shoulder. "Sorry to interrupt," she said. "But when you get to the part about calling a doctor, I'm right here."

Through the crowd she pushes... "Stand back, stand back," she commands. "I'm from the local surgery." The prostrate man breathes a weak sigh of relief, before she continues. "I'm the doctor's receptionist – the doctor can see you in two weeks' time. In the meantime, can you give be a brief description of your symptoms?"

All the organs of the body were having a meeting, trying to decide who was in charge.

The brain said: "I should be in charge, because I run all the body's systems, so without me nothing would happen."

"I should be in charge," said the heart, "because I pump the blood and circulate oxygen all over the body, so without me you'd all waste away."

"I should be in charge," said the stomach, "because I process food and give all of you energy."

"I should be in charge," said the rectum, "because I'm responsible for waste removal."

All the other body parts laughed at the rectum and insulted him, so in a huff, he shut down tight. Within a few days, the brain had a terrible headache, the stomach was bloated, and the blood was toxic. Eventually the other organs gave in. They all agreed that the rectum should be the boss. The moral of the story? You don't have to be smart or important to be in charge... just an arsehole.

Having lunch one day, a sex therapist said to her patient, "According to a survey we just completed, ninety percent of all people masturbate in the shower. Only ten percent of them sing."
"Really?" asked the patient.
The therapist nodded and proceeded to ask, "And do you know what song they sing?"
The patient shook her head and replied, "No."
The therapist replied, "I didn't think so."

Two guys were at the end of a bar when a young woman seated a table behind them began to choke on a sandwich. She was turning blue and was obviously having serious breathing difficulties. One of the guys turned to the other and said, "That girl is in big trouble! I reckon I should go and help."
He rushed over to her and asked "Madam, can you speak?" Still choking, she shook her head. So he said, "Listen darling. Can you breathe?" Again she shook her head. "Ok," he said, "brace yourself sweetheart!"
With that, he pulls up her skirt and licks her right on the butt. Completely shocked, the young woman coughs up the obstruction and amazingly begins to breathe normally again. The guy returns to his friend, who greets him, saying "ain't it funny how that hind-lick manoeuvre always does the trick."

> *What's grey, sits at the end of your bed and takes the piss out of you?*
> *A kidney dialysis machine.*

My memory's not a sharp as it used to be
(Also, my memory's not as sharp as it used to be)

> *"Can you give me something to lower my sex drive, please?"* an elderly man asked his GP.
> *"But surely at your age it's all in the mind,"* said the doctor.
> *"Yes,"* agreed the old man. *"That's why I need it lowered."*

Bert made an appointment with a urologist, famous for his work in the field of impotence. The doctor examined him and said, "You're in remarkably good condition for a man of 85. Why are you here?"

Bert replied, "My friend Arthur says he has sex twice a week. There's no way I could manage that."

The doctor shrugged. "Oh yes you can. You can certainly say you have sex as many times a week as you like."

An eminent doctor was giving a talk to the general public on the dangers of an unhealthy diet. He listed the dangers of high salt content, excessive sugar and unsaturated fats and ended by asking, "But do you know the one food that creates the most problems in life, one that we all either have eaten or are very likely to eat?"

The audience remained silent, until an elderly man suggested, "Wedding cake?"

At an old people's home an 88-year-old woman finished her dinner, stood up, held a clenched fist in the air and proclaimed: "Anyone who can guess what I have in my hand can have their wicked way with me tonight." It was met with silence.
"Come on, come on have a guess," she exhorted.
"An elephant!" called out one disinterested old duffer.
"Near enough," she replied.

> *The doctor placed a stethoscope on an elderly and slightly deaf female patient's anterior chest wall. "Big breaths," he instructed.*
> *"Well, they used to be," replied the patient.*

An old man went to the doctor complaining of a terrible pain in his leg. "I am afraid it's just old age," replied the doctor, "there is nothing that can be done about it." "Are you sure?" fumed the old man. "There's surely something you can do?"
"Ahh! You know better of course." snorted the doctor.
"Well it seems a matter of logic to me," the old man replied,
"My other leg is fine, and it's the exact same age!"

How do resistant bacterial strains thank each other in France? MRSi!

A man goes to visit his 85-year-old grandpa in hospital.
"How are you grandpa?" he asks.
"Feeling fine," says the old man.
"What's the food like?"
"Great! Really tasty."
"And the nursing?"
"Just couldn't be better. These young nurses really take care of you."
"What about sleeping? Do you sleep OK?"
"No problem, nine hours solid every night. At 10 o'clock they bring me a cup of hot chocolate and a Viagra tablet ... and that's it. I go out like a light."
The grandson is puzzled and a little alarmed by this, so rushes off to question the nurse in charge.
"What are you people doing?" he demands.
"He says you're giving an 85-year-old Viagra on a daily basis. Surely that can't be true?"
"Oh, yes. That's right," replies the nurse. "Every night at 10 o'clock we give him a cup of hot chocolate and a Viagra tablet. It works a treat. The chocolate makes him sleep, and the Viagra stops him from rolling out of bed."

When my wife finally awoke from her coma in the hospital this morning, I decided to give her the good news first.
"Darling, the doctors say you're going to pull through."
"Tell me the bad news," she whispered.
"You've failed your driving test."

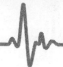

Three elderly men are at the doctor's office undergoing a senility test.
He asks the first man, "What is three times three?"
"274," he replies.
The doctor rolls his eyes and looks up at the ceiling, and asks the second man, "OK. How about you? Do you know what three times three is?"
"Tuesday," replies the second man.
The doctor shakes his head sadly, then asks the third man, "Fine. Your turn mister. What's three times three?"
"Nine," says the third man.
"Eureka!" says the doctor. "Now tell me. How did you get that?"
"Simple," he says, "I just subtracted 274 from Tuesday."

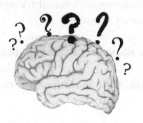

An elderly male resident of the nursing home said to the female resident in a wheelchair, "I bet you can't guess how old I am."
She replied, "I can if you take off all of your clothes."
So he stripped off completely and she instructed him to turn around slowly.
Then she said, "You're 95!"
"That's amazing!!" he exclaimed. "How could you tell?"
"You told me at breakfast."

At a nursing home, a group of senior citizens were sitting around talking about their aches and pains.

"My arms are so weak I can hardly lift this cup of coffee," said one.

"I know what you mean. My cataracts are so bad, I can't even see my coffee," replied another.

"I can't turn my head because of the arthritis in my neck," said a third, to which several nodded weakly in agreement.

"My blood pressure pills make me dizzy," another contributed.

"I guess that's what happens when we get old," sighed an old man as he slowly shook his head.

Then there was a short moment of silence.

"Well, it's not that bad," said one woman cheerfully. "At least we can all still drive."

> *The doctor was giving an octogenarian his annual check-up. "How do you feel, Albert?" said the doctor. "You're 85 now – that's some achievement. But are you OK?"*
> *"To be honest, Doc" said the old timer, "I feel like a new born babe."*
> *"Really?"*
> *"Yep. I've got no hair, no teeth, and I just peed myself."*

An 86-year-old man went to his doctor for his quarterly check-up.

The doctor asked him how he was feeling, and the 86-year-old said, "Things are great and I've never felt better."

I now have a 20 year-old bride who is pregnant with my child. "So what do you think about that Doc?"

The doctor considered his question for a minute and then began to tell a story.

"I have an older friend, much like you, who is an avid hunter and never misses a season."

One day he was setting off to go hunting. In a bit of a hurry, he accidentally picked up his walking cane instead of his gun."

"As he neared a lake, he came across a very large male deer sitting by the water's edge.

Suddenly he realized that he'd left his gun at home and so he couldn't shoot the magnificent creature. Instead, he raised his cane, aimed it at the animal pretending it was his good ol' hunting rifle and shouted 'bang, bang'.

"Incredibly, two shots rang out and the deer fell over dead. Now, what do you think of that?" asked the doctor.

The 86-year-old said, "Well, you would naturally assume that somebody else had shot a couple of rounds into that deer."

The doctor replied, "My point exactly."

An 85-year-old man went to the health clinic for his physical exam. When he finished, the doctor gave the man a jar saying he would need to do a sperm count.

"Take this jar home," he said "And bring back a semen sample tomorrow."

The next day the 85-year-old man reappeared at the doctor's office and gave him the jar, which was as clean and empty as on the previous day. The doctor asked what happened and the man explained,

"Well, doc, it's an odd thing. First I tried with my right hand, but nothing. Then I tried with my left hand, but still nothing. So I asked my wife to help me. She tries with her right hand, then with her left, but still nothing. She tried with her mouth, first with the teeth in, then with her teeth out. Again, still nothing."

"We even called up her friend Ethel and she tried too, first with both hands, then an armpit - and she even tried squeezing it between her knees, but as you can see – it was all to no avail."
The doctor was shocked. "What! You asked your neighbour?"

The old man replied, "Yep. Sorry but none of us could get the jar open."

One day a family brings their frail, elderly mother to an old people's home. They are concerned, but feel reassured that she is in good hands.

The next morning, the nurses bathe her, feed her a hearty breakfast and set her in a chair at a window overlooking a beautiful garden.

She seems fine, but after a while she slowly starts to lean over sideways in her chair.

Two attentive nurses immediately rush up to catch her and straighten her up.

Again there seems little wrong, but after a while she starts to tilt to the other side.

The nurses rush back and once more bring her back upright.

This dance continues all morning.

Later the family arrive to see how the old woman is getting on in her new home.

"So Mummy, how are you getting on here? Are they treating you well?" they ask.

"Oh yes," she replies. "It's all very nice." Then lowering her voice, she whispers, "Except they won't let me fart."

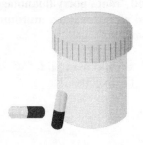

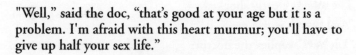

An 80-year-old man was having his annual physical. As the doctor put the stethoscope to his heart, he began muttering, "Uh oh!"

The man asked the doctor what the problem was.

"Well," said the doc, "it appears you have a serious heart murmur. Do you smoke?"

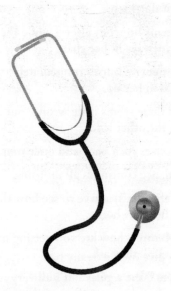

"Never have", replied the man.

"Do you drink in excess?

"I'm teetotal," replied the man.

"Do you have a sex life?"

"Oh yes, you bet!"

"Well," said the doc, "that's good at your age but it is a problem. I'm afraid with this heart murmur; you'll have to give up half your sex life."

Looking perplexed, the old man said, "Which half... the LOOKING or the THINKING?"

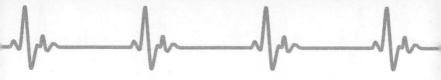

A man goes to his doctor and says, "I don't think my wife's hearing is as good as it used to be. What should I do?"

The doctor replies," Try this test and you'll find out for sure. When your wife is in the kitchen doing the dishes, stand five yards behind her and ask her a question. If she doesn't respond keep moving closer repeating the question until she hears you."

The man goes home and sees his wife preparing dinner. He stands five yards behind her and says, "What's for dinner, honey?" He gets no response, so he moves to three yards behind her and asks again. There is still no response, so he moves a yard nearer. Still nothing. Finally he stands directly behind her and repeats, "Honey, what's for dinner?"

She replies, "For the fourth time, I SAID CHICKEN!"

A seventy-year man goes to the doctor for a health check-up. After some tests and checks, the doctor comes in with a grave look on his face. He says:

"Well, I have some bad news and some really bad news."

The patient is shocked:

"Well, give me the really bad news first," he says.

The doc takes a gulp and bleats out the awful news:

"You have cancer, and only 6 months to live."

The man is clearly shocked.

"And there's worse news, doc?"

"Uh huh," replies the doctor:

"You also have Alzheimer's disease."

"Thank God," the man answers. "I was afraid I had cancer!"

An old man suffering from diarrhoea and urinary incontinence goes to the doctor. The doctor asks for a number of samples and asks the patient to return the next day with the specimen bottles. The old man is a little confused, but collects all the little jars and goes home. At home, the worried man not knowing how he's going to fill all these bottles in one day explains to his wife that the doctor had requested stool, urine, and semen samples.

His wife however seems to take it all in her stride.

"That's easy," she says, relief obvious in her voice. "All he wants is your pyjama trousers."

"Ah! Mr Brockley," said the GP to his elderly patient. "What brings you to my surgery on this fine spring morning? The arthritis playing up again?"

"No Doc that's all fine at the moment. It's a slightly more delicate matter."

"Uh-huh. The old plumbing not what it was eh?"

"No Doc, that's fine too. But I need your help. You see every time I make love to my wife I get these dizzy spells, my legs go weak and I find it really hard to catch my breath."

"Well Mr Brockley, it comes to us all with age I'm afraid. But I'll see what I can do. Now tell me, when did you first notice these symptoms?"

The old man looked up and replied "Well it happened three times last night and twice this morning."

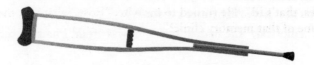

Two old ladies were outside their nursing home, having a smoke, when it started to rain. One of the ladies pulled out a condom, cut off the end, put it over her cigarette, and continued smoking.

"What's that?" asked the first old lady.

"A condom. This way my cigarette doesn't get wet." replied the second.

Obviously impressed, her friend asked "Where did you get it?"

"You can get them at any chemist." said the second little old lady.

The next day, the first old lady hobbled into the local chemist and announced to the pharmacist that she wanted a packet of condoms.

The man looked at her strangely (she was, after all, over 80 years of age), but politely asked what brand she preferred.

"It doesn't matter," she answered, "as long as it fits a Camel."

Two elderly couples were enjoying friendly conversation when one of the men asked the other, "Fred, how was the memory clinic you went to last month?"

"Outstanding," Fred replied. "They taught us all the latest psychological techniques: visualization, association, etc. It was great."

"That's super!" His friend retorted. "I might even try it myself. What was the name of the clinic?"

Fred went blank. He thought and thought, but couldn't remember. Then a smile broke across his face and he asked, "What do you call that flower with the long stem and thorns?"

"You mean a rose?"

"Yes, that's it!" He turned to his wife, "Rose, what was the name of that memory clinic?"

At the bar of the local pub the conversation turned to the pros and cons of various ways of preserving health. One stout elderly man held forth with great eloquence on the subject.

"Look at me!" he said. "Never a day's sickness in my life, and all due to simple food. Why, gentlemen," he continued, "from the age of twenty to that of forty I lived an absolutely simple regular life – no fancy foods, no late hours, no extravagances. Every day, in fact, summer and winter, I was in bed regularly at nine o'clock and up again at five in the morning. I worked from eight to one, then had dinner – a plain dinner, mark: after that, an hour's exercise; then…"

At this point an impatient stranger in the corner, butted in. "Excuse me, sir," he asked, "but what were you inside for?"

> A 70-year-old man sat down in the orthopaedic surgeon's office. "You know, Doc," he said, "I've made love in more exotic cars than anyone I know. Must be at least a thousand."
> "And now, I suppose, you want me to treat you for the arthritis you got from scrunching up in all those uncomfortable positions," the doctor said.
> "Heck, no," the old fellow replied. "I want to borrow your Lamborghini."

One day two elderly women and an old gentleman were sitting in a full waiting room. The two old women were talking to each other while the old man just sat there between them staring at the floor. Then in a very loud voice, one lady said to the other while pointing to the frail old man sitting between them, "He has aids you know." Now, as everybody in the waiting room was staring at the poor old gent, she continued, saying, "but he forgot to put them in this morning."

Doctor to an elderly, obviously distressed patient:
"No Mrs Smith, not a HEARSE, I'm calling for a NURSE!"

An older man is on the operating table awaiting surgery. He has insisted that his son, a renowned surgeon, perform the operation. He is about to receive the anesthesia when he asks to speak to his son.
"Yes, Dad, what is it?"
"Listen son, don't be nervous, do your best. Oh, and just remember, if it doesn't go well, if something happens to me, your mother is going to come and live with you and your wife."

An elderly patient went to have her teeth checked.
"Mrs McNamee, your teeth are good for the next 50 years," the dentist beamed.
To which she replied, "Oh goodness gracious. What will they do without me?"

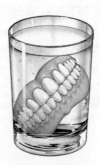

An elderly gentleman went to see his doctor and asked for a prescription of Viagra. The doctor said,
"That's no problem. How many do you want?"
The man answered,
"Just a few, maybe 4, but cut each one in 4 pieces."
The doctor said, "That won't do you any good. I don't think that much will help you have sex."
The elderly gentleman said, "That's alright. I don't need them for sex anymore. I am over 90 years old for God's sake. I just want my dick to stick out far enough so I don't pee on my shoes."

An elderly woman went into the doctor's office. When the doctor asked why she was there, she replied, "I'd like to have some birth-control pills." Taken aback, the doctor thought for a minute and then said,

"Excuse me, Mrs Smith, but you're 72 years old. What possible use could you have for birth control pills?"

The woman responded, "They help me sleep better."

The doctor thought some more and continued, "How in the world do birth control pills help you to sleep?"

The woman said, "It's simple, I put them in my granddaughter's orange juice every morning and I sleep a whole lot better at night."

> *Patient:* *I have yellow teeth, what do I do?*
>
> *Dentist:* *Wear a brown tie.*

When the doctor called Mrs Godfrey to tell her that her cheque came back, she replied, "Isn't that strange. So did my arthritis!"

An old woman stopped me in the street and asked me to show her how to get to the hospital. So I pushed her under a bus.

> *A GP was taking the details of a new elderly patient, who had been added to his lists. "How long have you been bedridden?" he asked. After a look of complete confusion she answered, "Why, not for about twenty years - when my husband was still alive."*

An older gentleman had lost his hearing aid and wanted to get a new one. Before getting the new hearing aid, he wanted his ear cleaned out, so he went to his doctor.

As the doctor was cleaning his ears, he noticed a foreign object lodged in the man's ear canal. With a pair a tweezers, the doctor removed the object. Upon closer examination, he discovered that it was a suppository. The doctor told the older gentleman that he had a suppository stuck in his ear.

At this, the man exclaimed,

"Now I know where I put my hearing aid!"

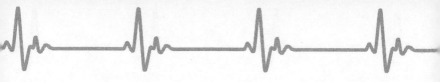

Mr Murphy was an old man with Alzheimer's who lived in a nursing home. One day he came out of his room, tracked down the nearest nurse, and said,

"My penis is dead!"

The nurse kindly replied, "I'm sorry to hear that, Mr. Murphy, but it happens all the time with men your age."

The very next day, Mr Murphy came out of his room with his penis sticking out of his pants and wandered up and down the hall. The same nurse saw him and said, "Mr Murphy, I thought you told me that your penis was dead."

He said, "I did – but today is the viewing."

Three old men were sitting around and talking. The 80 year-old said, "The best thing that could happen to me would just to be able to have a good pee. I stand there for twenty minutes, and it dribbles and hurts. I have to go over and over again."

The 85 year-old said, "The best thing that could happen to me is if I could have one good bowel movement. I take every kind of laxative I can get my hands on and it's still a problem."

Then the 90 year-old said, "That's not my problem. Every morning at 6:00 am sharp, I have a good long pee. At around 6:30 am I have a great bowel movement. The best thing that could happen to me would be if I could wake up before 7:00 am.

A 47-year-old man has a face-lift for his birthday. On his way home from the clinic he pops into the newsagent to buy a paper. Before leaving he says to the newsagent, "I hope you don't mind me asking, but how old do you think I am?" "About 35," comes the reply.
"I'm actually 47 years old," the man says, feeling really happy.

Next he goes into the fish and chip shop and, again, before leaving he asks the same question, to which the reply is, "Oh, you look about 29." This makes the man feel really good.

Then as he is standing at a bus stop he asks an old woman the same question.
She replies, "I'm 85 years old and my eyesight is going. But when I was young there was a sure way of telling a man's age. If I put my hand down your trousers and play with your wedding tackle for ten minutes I will be able to tell your exact age."

The man thinks 'What the hell' and lets her slip her hand down his trousers.

Ten minutes later the old lady announces, "You're 47 years old." Stunned, the man says, "That was brilliant. How did you do that?"

The old lady replies, "Well to be honest – I was behind you in the chip shop."

58

An elderly man visits his doctor as he is no longer able to perform sexually. "I've tried Viagra, Doc but it does nothing.

"Is there anything else you can give me?"

The doctor replies "I really shouldn't do this, I could be struck off. But go to this address and ask for Mrs Jacobs. Tell her I sent you for 'The Special'.

The man does as he says and calls at the address. The woman rubs some strange herbal ointment on his privates and tells him, "Listen carefully. This is powerful stuff and you can only use it once. All you have to do is say '123' and your member shall rise for as long as you wish!"

The man then asks, "What happens when I'm through, and I don't want to continue?" The woman replies, "When your partner is completely exhausted and can take no more sex, all she has to say is '1234', and it will then go down. But be warned; choose your moment wisely for you will not be able to repeat the trick."

That night the old man slides into bed, cuddles up to his wife and says "123". As promised he suddenly has the most gigantic erection ever. This is fantastic, he thinks, wondering how long he can keep it going... Then his wife turns over and asks, "What did you say '123' for?"

Medical College
a font of knowledge, here all go to drink

A doctor was giving a lecture to a group of medical students at the local hospital. Pointing to the x-ray, he explained:
"As you can see, this patient limps because his right fibula and tibia are radically arched."
The doctor looked up at the assembled students, and asked one of them: "Now what would you do in a case like this?"
The student replied: "I suppose I would limp too."

Two medical students were walking along the street when they saw an old man walking with his legs spread apart. He was stiff-legged and walking slowly.
One student said to his friend: "I'm sure that poor old man has Burgess Syndrome. Those people walk just like that."
The other student says: "No, I don't think so. The old man surely has Dubrisky Syndrome. He walks slowly and his legs are apart just as we learned in class."
Since they couldn't agree they decided to ask the old man. They approached him and one of the students said to him: "We're medical students and couldn't help but notice the way you walk, but we couldn't agree on the syndrome you might have. Could you tell us what it is?"
The old man said, "I'll tell you, but first you tell me what you two fine medical students think."
The first student said, "I think its Burgess Syndrome."
The old man said, "You thought....... but you are wrong."
The other student said, "I think you have Dubrisky Syndrome."
The old man said, "You thought....... but you are wrong.
So they asked him, "Well, old timer, what do you have?"
The old man said, "I thought it was a fart........
but I was wrong, too!"

First year medical students were receiving their first anatomy class with a cadaver. They all gathered around the table with the body covered with a white sheet. The professor started the class by telling them:

"In medicine, it is necessary to have two important qualities: the first is that you can not be disgusted by anything involving the human body."

For an example, the professor pulled back the sheet, stuck his finger in the anus of the corpse, and withdrew it. To his students dismay he then took his finger and stuck it in his mouth.

"Now I'd like you all to go ahead and do the same thing."

The students hesitated for several minutes, but eventually took turns sticking a finger in the anus of the corpse and sucking on it. When everyone finished, the professor looked at them and told them:

"The second most important quality in a doctor is observation. Any observant students would have noticed that I stuck in my middle finger but sucked on my index finger. Now learn to pay attention."

An applicant was being interviewed for admission to a famous medical school.

"Tell me," inquired the interviewer, "where do you expect to be in ten years time?"

"Well, let's see," replied the student. "It's Wednesday afternoon so I guess that I'll be on the golf course by now."

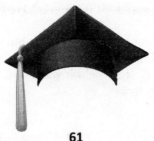

> *A skeleton escapes the medical
> college and heads for a bar.
> He says, "Gimme a beer... and a mop."*

The medical student was asked four reasons why mother's milk
was better for babies than cow's milk.
This is the answer he submitted:

1. It's fresher.
2. It's cleaner.
3. The cats can't get to it.
4. It's easier to take on a picnic.

He then added: "It also comes in such cute containers."

A Brief History of Medicine

I have an earache....

2000 B.C. Here, eat this root.
1000 A.D. That root is heathen, say this prayer.
1850 A.D. That prayer is superstition, drink this potion.
1940 A.D. That potion is snake oil, swallow this pill.
1985 A.D. That pill is ineffective, take this antibiotic.
2000 A.D. That antibiotic is artificial. Here, eat this root...

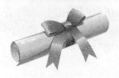

Back at the Doc's

What did the doctor say to the dwarf?
You've got hi-ho hi-ho high-ho blood pressure!

I went to my doctor to ask for something for persistent wind. He gave me a kite.

A man had a problem getting up in the morning. He was always getting in trouble for being late for work. After being given one last warning before being sacked, he decided to go to the doctor. His GP was very understanding and prescribed a difficult-to-pronounce pill. After taking the pill that night, the man slept soundly, and woke in plenty of time to get ready for work. "Morning!" he announced, checking his watch on his arrival. "At last I really think my timekeeping worries are over." His boss however didn't look so happy. "That's great," he replied. "But where were you yesterday?"

A man goes to the doctor about his painful ear.
"I'm sure I've got something stuck in there, Doc," he complains. The GP gets out his auriscope and has a good look.
"You're dead right," he mumbles. Getting out his tweezers he slowly extracts a fifty pound note from the man's ear.
"Hold on," he exclaims as the man starts to get up, "there's more." Slowly he begins to pull a load more fifties along with lots of tens and fives. Finally when he had removed all the notes, the doctor counted up the money – one thousand, nine hundred and ninety five pounds.
"Well, that explains it," announced the patient.
"I knew I wasn't feeling two grand."

A man went to the doctor with a tiny green pimple on his face. The doc prescribed some cream, but a week later it had grown into a small shoot.

"Keep using the cream," advised the puzzled medic but by the next week a tree was clearly growing out of the patient's head.

"Double the dosage," bluffed the baffled GP. Within a month, the man's whole head was covered by trees, a park, a stream and picnic tables.

"Ah now I see the problem," exclaimed the relieved doctor. "You've grown a beauty spot!"

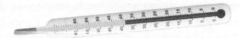

A man hasn't been feeling well, so he goes to his doctor for a complete check up. Afterwards, the doctor comes out with the results.

"I'm afraid I have some very bad news," the doctor says. "You're dying, and you don't have much time left."

"Oh, that's terrible!" says the man. "Give it to me straight, Doc. How long have I got?"

"Ten," the doctor says sadly.

"Ten?" the man asks. "Ten what? Months? Weeks? What?"

"Nine, eight..."

"Doctor please help me, my wife thinks she's a satellite dish."

"Don't worry Mr Jones, I can cure her."

"I don't want her cured Doc; I just want you to adjust her so I can get Sky Sports.

A man went to the doctor complaining that every time he spoke, he farted. "You must help me, Doc. It's extremely embarrassing. The only saving grace is that the farts don't smell."

"True enough, his every word was accompanied by a noise like someone was stepping on a duck.

"Hmm!" said the doctor, "I'll have to send you to a specialist."

"Will that be a gastro-enterologist or a surgeon?" said the patient.

"Neither," said the doctor. "I'm sending you to an Ear, Nose & Throat specialist. If you think those farts don't smell, then you've got something wrong with your nose!"

"Doctor, doctor, I feel like a moth."

"You should visit a psychologist."

"I was on my way there but I noticed your light was on."

"Doctor, doctor, I keep getting this urge to sing "The green, green grass of home".

"Clearly you have a touch of Tom Jones-itus."

"Crikey, is it a common condition?"

"It's not unusual..."

A paper bag walks into a GP, complaining of headaches and generally feeling run down. The GP runs a few tests and calls him back for the results.

The doctor says "I'm really sorry, but you appear to have a rare genetic condition. It's quite serious."

"But doc, how?? I'm just a paper bag!"

"I'm afraid your father must have been a carrier."

A man had just undergone a physical examination and the doctor was explaining his rather extensive prescription: Take green pill with a glass of water after getting up. Take blue pill with glass of water after lunch. Just before bed take red pill with another glass of water.

"Doctor," the patient pleaded. "Give it to me straight. What exactly is wrong with me?"

The doc looked him in the eye and said "You're not getting enough water."

"Doctor, Doctor, I keep thinking I'm the school bell."

"Take these tablets and if they don't work give me a ring in the morning."

A man walks into a doctor's office. He has a cucumber up his nose, a carrot in his left ear and a banana in his right ear.

"What's the matter with me?" he asks the doctor.

The doctor replies, "You're not eating properly."

Doctor! I have a serious problem; I can never remember what I just said.
When did you first notice this problem?
What problem?

The Doctor said he needed to operate on my funny bone. In next to no time, he had me in stitches.

"Impotence," explained the doctor, "is just nature's way of saying, 'no hard feelings'."

Overheard in a GP's surgery:

Doctor: Are you on HRT?
Patient: No, Income Support.

My doctor asked me *"Are you on the BBC Diet?"*
So I asked him," *What's the BBC Diet?"*
He said, *"BBC. Buy Bigger Clothes."*

A man goes to the doctor. "I think I'm a Tyrannosaurus Rex," he says.
"Hmm," says the Doc. "Open wide and say 'Ahh', please."
The dinosaur opens his mouth as wide as he can and says "Raaaaar!"
"Good, good. Now stand and touch your toes," says the Doc.
"Are you taking the piss?" says the T Rex. "With these arms?"

"Doctor, Doctor, I'm becoming invisible."

Yes I can see you're not all there!

A woman visited her doctor for the fifth time that month.
"You better face it," the doctor told her. "You're suffering from hypochondria."
"Oh no, not that as well!" replied the woman.

Patient: It's been one month since my last visit and I still feel pretty awful.
Doctor: Did you follow the instructions on the medicine I gave you?
Patient: I sure did – the bottle said 'keep tightly closed.

A young doctor is staying at a hotel in the West of Ireland during a medical conference. Coming home one night, he finds an agitated hotel owner waiting for him.
"Doctor!" he cries. "We've found some bones in one of the walls. Can you come and tell us if they are human?"
The doctor is led down to the cellar, where builders have begun to remove part of the wall. They had stopped when a small cavity had been discovered with some bones inside. The doctor pulls some of the bricks away to reveal a full skeleton. Dangling around the shoulders is a gold medallion, inscribed with the words: 'Irish Hide-and-Seek Champion 1927'.

A man calls his doctor and frantically says, "Doctor, I think my wife is dead!"

The doctor replies, "What do you mean you 'think' she's dead?"

Well doctor," says the man, "the sex is the same, but the dishes are piling up in the sink."

"Doctor, Doctor, you told me not to worry about my son wetting his bed at night and that it's perfectly normal. Well I've thought about it and I'm really not so sure – and neither is his wife!"

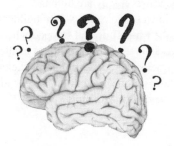

The Miracle of Childbirth

Little Johnny's neighbours had a baby. Unfortunately the baby was born without ears. When the mother and new baby came home from the hospital, Johnny's family was invited over to see the baby.

Before they left their house, Little Johnny's dad had a talk with him and explained that the baby had no ears. His dad also told him that if he so much as mentioned anything about the baby's missing ears or even said the word 'ears' he would get the beating of his life when they came back home. Little Johnny told his dad he understood completely.

When Johnny looked in the cot he said, "What a beautiful baby."

The mother said, "Why, thank you, Little Johnny."

Johnny said, "He has beautiful little feet and beautiful little hands, a cute little nose and really beautiful eyes. Can he see ok?"

"Yes, the mother replied, we are so thankful. The doctor said he will have 20/20 vision."

"That's great," said Little Johnny, "because he'd be stuffed if he needed glasses."

> *Not long after my wife had given birth,*
> *I asked the doctor,*
> *"How soon do you think we'll be able to have sex?"*
> *He smiled at me and said,*
> *"I'm off duty in ten minutes –*
> *meet me in the car park."*

A woman gives birth to a baby. Afterwards the doctor comes into the room and says,
"I have something to tell you about your child ..."
The woman slowly sits up with a worried look on her face and says, "What's wrong with it?"
The doctor says, "There's nothing really wrong with it, it's just a little different! It's a hermaphrodite."
The woman looks confused. "A hermaphrodite, what's that?"
The doctor replies, "It has both features of a male and a female."
The woman looks relieved. "What? You mean it has a penis and a brain?"

Brenda, pregnant with her first child, was paying a visit to her obstetrician's office. When the exam was over, she shyly began, "My husband wants me to ask you..."

"I know, I know." the doctor said, placing a reassuring hand on her shoulder, "I get asked that all the time. Sex is fine until late in the pregnancy."

"No, that's not it at all," Brenda confessed. "He wants to know if I can still mow the lawn."

A married couple went to the hospital to have their baby delivered. Upon their arrival, the doctor said he had invented a new machine that would transfer a percentage of the mother's labour pain to the father.

He asked if they were willing to try it out. The husband took some persuading, but his wife said it was the least he could do considering what she had to go through. So the doctor set the pain transfer to 10% for starters, explaining that even 10% was probably more pain than the father had ever experienced before. But as the labour progressed, the husband felt fine and asked the doctor to go ahead and kick it up a notch. The doctor then adjusted the machine to 20% pain transfer. The husband was still feeling fine – women had obviously made too much of this childbirth pain.

The doctor checked the husband's blood pressure and was amazed at how well he was doing. At this point they decided to try for 50%. The husband continued to feel quite well. Since the pain transfer was obviously helping out the wife considerably, the husband encouraged the doctor to transfer all the pain to him. The wife delivered a healthy baby with virtually no pain. She and her husband were ecstatic.

When they got home, the postman lay dead on the drive.

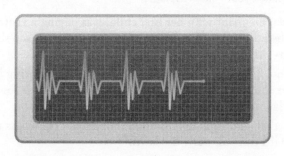

One day, Mr Tipton rushed his pregnant wife over to the hospital. As the doctors were prepping his wife, Mrs Tipton's brother Wayne arrived to be there to congratulate his sister. The birth went ahead fine with Mrs Tipton giving birth to two healthy twins. However when Mr Tipton saw the afterbirth, he fainted and cracked open his head.

Later Mr. Tipton woke up in a bed with the doctor standing above him.

"Mr Tipton," the doctor said, "we've performed surgery and you are going to be fine."

"But what about my wife – and the babies," he said, suddenly remembering.

"Don't worry, your wife is fine and so are the twins," replied the surgeon. "You have a handsome boy and a beautiful baby girl. And they're already named! Because you were unconscious and your wife was still under anaesthesia, she requested that her brother Wayne name the kids."

"No! Her brother! He's a complete idiot? I can't believe she let him! Oh my God, what did he name them?"

"He named your daughter Denise," relayed the surgeon.

"Hey, not bad! Perhaps I underestimated my brother-in-law. What did he name my son?"

"He named your son Denephew."

In the backwoods of Scotland, Davey's wife went into labour in the middle of the night, and the doctor was called out to assist in the delivery. To keep the nervous father-to-be busy, the doctor handed him a lantern and said:

"Here lad, you hold this high so I can see what I'm doing."
Soon, a wee baby boy was brought into the world.

"Whoa there sonny!" said the doctor. "Don't be in a rush to put the lantern down... I think there's another wee one to come yet."
Sure enough, within minutes he had delivered a bonnie lass.

"No, no, don't be in a great hurry to be putting down that lantern, lad... it seems there's another one on the way!" cried the doctor.
Then the man scratched his head in bewilderment, and asked the doctor: "Do ye think it's the light that's attracting them?"

A woman goes to her doctor who confirms that she is pregnant. As this is her first pregnancy, the doctor checks whether she has any questions.

"Well, I'm a little worried about the pain," she replies, "how much will it hurt when I finally give birth?"

The doctor answers, "Well, it does vary from woman to woman and pregnancy to pregnancy and as is commonly debated in the medical profession, it's difficult to rate pain."

"I understand, but can't you give me a vague idea?" she asks.

"I'll have a try," replies the doc. "If you grab your upper lip and pull it out a little..." She does what he asks. "Good, but try pulling it a little more..."

She stretches it a little more. "Like this?" she asks.

"No. A little more..."

This carries on until she is clearly in some discomfort.

It is only at that point the doctor tells her, "Now stretch it over your head!"

A young lady had just visited her doctor and he informed her that she was pregnant. The young lady had been married for ten years and had wanted a baby very badly. As she sat on the bus on her way home, she felt that she had to share the good news with someone. The gentleman sitting next to her seemed as good as anyone to tell.

Sir, she said, I just received the best news you could ever imagine. I have to share it with someone or I'll bust. Then she told him how she had been desperate to get pregnant and thought it would never happen but now the doctor had told her she was finally pregnant.

The man listened and nodded. "I know exactly how you feel," he told her. He said he was a farmer and he had great trouble getting his hens to lay. He tried all different feeds and drugs but to no avail. Then one morning he went out to the hen house and all of his hens had laid eggs. He was so happy. Then, with a smile, he added, "but confidentially, I changed cocks."

The newly pregnant woman looked him back in the eye and whispered, "Confidentially, me too."

A woman and a baby were in the GP's room, waiting for the doctor to come in for the baby's first exam. The doctor arrived and examined the baby, checked his weight, and being a little concerned, asked if the baby was breast-fed or bottle-fed. "Breast-fed," she replied.

"Well, strip down to your waist," the doctor ordered. She did. He pinched her nipples, pressed, kneaded, and rubbed both breasts for a while in a very professional and detailed examination. Motioning to her to get dressed, the doctor said, "No wonder this baby is underweight. You don't have any milk."

"I know," she said, "I'm his Grandma, but I'm glad I came."

A woman starts dating a married doctor. Soon she reveals that she is pregnant and both parties are unhappy with the situation. So the Doc dreams up a cunning plan.

"Don't worry," he says. "I work in the hospital. I'll find a solution."

About nine months later, at the same time as the woman goes in to give birth, a priest goes into the same hospital for a prostate operation. The doctor says to the woman,

"Here's the plan. After I've operated on the priest, I'll give the baby to him and tell him it was a miracle."

"Sounds unlikely but I suppose it's worth a try." she says. So the doctor delivers the baby and then operates on the priest.

After the operation he goes in to the priest and says,

"Father, you're not going to believe this."

"What?" asks the priest, "what happened?"

"You gave birth to a child!"

"But that's impossible!" says the priest.

"I just did the operation," insists the doctor, "it's a miracle! Here's your baby boy."

About 16 years go by, and the now ex-priest realizes he must tell his son the truth. One day, he sits the boy down and says,

"Son, I have something to tell you. I'm not your father."

The son is dismayed.

"What do you mean, you're not my father?"

The former priest replies,

"I am your mother. The archbishop is your father."

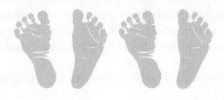

> *Did you hear about the baby born in the brand new high-tech delivery room?*
>
> *It was cordless!*

A father-to-be is pacing up and down at home while his wife is in hospital giving birth. The phone rings and the bloke answers.

"This is the hospital, sir; your wife has given birth to twins. However, there are more on the way."

The man puts the phone down and takes a large swig of vodka. The phone rings again.

"This is the hospital, your wife has had another little boy, and there are still more on the way."

The man drinks the whole bottle of vodka, by now he is totally drunk. He picks up the phone to ring the hospital to find out if she's had any more babies but, by mistake, he rings Lords Cricket Ground. When the phone is answered, he asks, "What's the latest?"

The person on the line replies,

"97 all out, and the last one was a duck!"

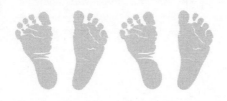

*When a hospital runs out of maternity nurses
do they call it a 'mid-wife crisis'?*

Don was seconds away from receiving a vasectomy when his brother and sister-in-law barged in the room holding their newborn baby."

Stop! You can't do this!" exclaimed the brother.

"And why not?" asked Don.

"Don't you want to have a beautiful baby someday like my wife and I have here?"

Don said nothing.

The brother grew impatient,

"C'mon Don, I want a nephew. Don, make me an uncle."

Don couldn't take it anymore. He gave his sister-in-law an apologetic look and asked his brother,

"You're absolutely sure you want a nephew?"

"Yes," the brother replied. "It would be an honour!"

"Well congratulations, you're holding him!"

Where does a test tube baby live?

Answer: In a womb with a view.

In Surgery
"Scalpel... Sutures... Clamp...
Whoops!... Pen... Death Certificate..."

A soldier goes into the hospital for surgery after being wounded in battle.

Waking up from the anaesthesia he sees his doctor standing at his bedside. "So tell me Doc, what did you do to me?"

The doctor says, "Son, we have some good news and some bad news."

"Yeah, what?" replies the patient.

"Well the good news is that we were able to save your private parts."

"Yes, that is good news Doc, but what about the bad news?"

"We put them under your pillow!"

The young man was quite adamant. He insisted to the surgeon that he wanted to be castrated. The surgeon pointed out that this was a drastic step for a young man to take and strongly urged him to reconsider his request.

"No," said the young man, "I have thought long and hard about it, I have read all there is about it and my mind is made up. I must have the operation."

The operation was duly carried out and when he had recovered from the anaesthetic and was back in the ward he got to talking to the other patients.

"And what are you in here for?" he asked the fellow in the next bed.

"To be circumcised." said his neighbour.

"Oh God!" screamed the young man, "that was the word I meant!"

Earlier this year Sam lost his ear in an unfortunate accident. The doctors tried to graft it back but the graft just wouldn't take. They were however prepared to try a radical new surgical experiment and replace it with a pig's ear. Once they had cut it to size, and sewn it in place, no one would be able to tell the difference, they claimed.

Sam went ahead with the operation and all seemed to go pretty well. But after a few weeks he was back at the surgery complaining bitterly that there was constant interference in his hearing and it was causing discomfort and migraines.

The doctors however were unwilling to hear criticism from their guinea pig. As far as they were concerned the pig ear transplant was a total success and he was just getting upset by a little bit of crackling.

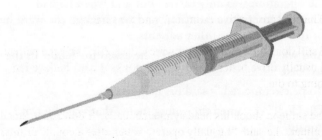

I went for an operation earlier to get rid of an infection in my ear. After waking up from the general anaesthetic the surgeon was very sympathetic. He told me that the operation had been a success but that I only had 18 months left.

I was shocked and stunned. How had things gone so wrong? So I asked how was it possible for a simple ear infection to cause a life to be cut short. What could have gone so badly wrong?"

How we both laughed when he explained
"No, no. I said 'You only have an ear and a half!"

The surgeon entered his patient's hospital room, ready to tell him the bad news.

"I hate to tell you this," he said, "but your internal injuries are severe. There is continuous bleeding, several organs have stopped functioning, and there is widespread infection. I did what I could in surgery, but you probably have less than twenty-four hours to live."

"Twenty-four hours!" said the patient, shaking his head.

"That's a conservative estimate," said the surgeon.

"I still don't understand how I wrecked my car," said the patient. "I usually drive better after a couple drinks. I can't believe I'm going to die."

The surgeon shook his head sympathetically. "I don't understand it either," he said. "I usually operate better after a couple drinks."

10 More Things You Don't Want to Hear During Surgery

🚑 Hmm... Let's try something new today!

🚑 Eughhh! Blood!!

🚑 Cool! Now can you make his leg twitch?

🚑 Are you completely sure this wasn't down as a vasectomy?

🚑 Anyone see where I left that scalpel?

🚑 I wish I hadn't forgotten my glasses.

🚑 Nurse, did this patient have an organ donor card?

🚑 Don't worry; I think it is sharp enough.

🚑 Damn! Someone's torn out page 96 of the manual!

🚑 Well folks, this will be a first for medical science.

Surgeon leaving operating room: That was close!
Assistant: What do you mean?
Surgeon: An inch either way or I would have been out of
     my specialty.

In the hospital, a patient's relatives gathered in the waiting room, where their family member lay gravely ill. Finally, the doctor came in looking tired and sombre.

"I'm afraid I am the bearer of bad news," he said as he surveyed the worried faces. "The only hope left for your loved one at this time is a brain transplant. It's an experimental procedure, semi-risky, and you will have to pay for the brain yourselves."

The family members sat silent as they absorbed the news. At last, someone asked,

"Well, how much does a brain cost?"

The doctor quickly responded,

"$200 for a female brain, and $500 for a male brain."

The moment turned awkward. Men in the room tried not to smile, avoiding eye contact with the women, but some actually smirked. A girl, unable to control her curiosity, blurted out the question everyone wanted to ask,

"Why is the male brain so much more?"

The doctor smiled at her childish innocence and then said,

"It's a standard pricing procedure. We have to mark the female brains down, because they're used!"

> *"The surgeon removed my left atrium and my left ventricle,"*
> *John said half-heartedly.*

The husband and wife agreed that they would tell no one about where the skin came from, and requested that the doctor also honour their secret.

After the surgery was completed, everyone was astounded at the woman's new beauty. She looked more beautiful than she ever had before! All her friends and relatives just went on and on about her youthful beauty!

One day, she was alone with her husband, and she was overcome with emotion at his sacrifice. She said, "Dear, I just want to thank you for everything you did for me. There is no way I could ever repay you."

"My darling," he replied, "Think nothing of it. I get all the thanks I need every time I see your mother kiss you on the cheek."

A man had a terrible accident. His manhood was mangled and torn from his body.

The doctor reassured him that modern medicine made it possible for his manhood to be rebuilt, but insurance didn't cover the expense. It was considered cosmetic.

He had three choices - small for £3,500, medium for £6,500 and large for £14,000.

The man was sure he'd want a medium or large. The doctor suggested that he discuss it with his wife privately before a final decision was made.

The doctor left the room and while he was gone the man called his wife and told her their options.

The doctor returned and found the man looking very sad.

"Did you make a decision?" the doctor asked.

"Yes," said the man. "She'd rather remodel the kitchen!"

A surgeon claims these are actual comments from his patients made while he was performing colonoscopies:

1. "Take it easy, Doc, you're boldly going where no man has gone before."

2. "Found Lord Lucan yet?"

3. "Can you hear me NOW?"

4. "You know, in some states of America, we're now legally married."

5. "Any sign of the trapped miners, Chief?"

6. "You put your left hand in, you take your left hand out. You do the Hokey Cokey..."

7. "Hey! Now I know how a Muppet feels!"

8. "Hey, Doc, let me know if you find my dignity."

9. "Could you write me a note for my wife, saying that my head is not, in fact, up there?"

10. "Don't tell me – I've got what my friends had been telling me I was for years... a perfect asshole."

11. "While you're there... My wife is missing a ring and I've misplaced a Custom Eldorado hot wheels toy."

Two little kids lined up for surgery are lying in stretchers outside the operating room.

The first kid leans over and asks,

"What are you in here for?"

The second kid says,

"I'm in here to get my tonsils out and I'm a little nervous."

The first kid tries to reassure the other and says,

"Oh! Don't worry. It's very simple. I had that done when I was four. They put you to sleep, and when you wake up they give you lots of ice cream and jelly."

The second kid, feeling a little better, then asks,

"What are you here for?"

The first kid says, "A circumcision."

The second kid says,

"Whoa! I had that done when I was born. I couldn't walk for a year!"

One surgeon to another: "Cultural differences aside, doctor, I wish you would stop referring to the patient's organs as giblets."

When his car mechanic came in for an operation, Dr Parker couldn't help but take the opportunity to turn the tables on him. "Well Mr 'Kwik-Exhaust'," said the doctor, "it's going to take at least five days for the parts to come in... And as for the cost, there's no way to tell until we get in there and see exactly what the problem."

A garage mechanic was removing a cylinder head from the engine of a Rolls Royce when he spotted a well-known heart surgeon. The mechanic called him over saying: "Hey, Doc, look at this engine. I open it up, take the valves out, mend them and put them back in, and when I finish, it works just like new. So how come I get paid a pittance and you get such a tasty salary? You and I are doing basically the same work."

The surgeon paused, smiled and leaned over, and said to the mechanic..." Try doing it with the engine running."

I was going to be a cardiologist, but I really didn't have the heart.

"What are my chances of living through this, doctor?"
"Well, I've done this operation 87 times..."
"Great, that's nice to know."
"...and I'm bound to get it right one of these days."

Overheard in the Ear, Nose and Throat department:

Impatient Surgeon: **For Heaven's sake nurse, get me my auriscope!**

Distraught young nurse: **But Doctor, I don't even know your star sign.**

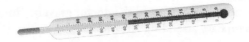

Three Doctors are at a convention talking shop.

The first Doctor says: "I love doing surgery on Artists, they are so colourful: red hearts, pink stomachs, green spleens."
The next Doctor says:
"Me, I love doing surgery on Accountants, open them up and all their parts are numbered, makes it very easy."
The third Doctor says:
"I love doing surgery on Lawyers, they have no heart, they have no guts and the head and the ass are interchangeable!"

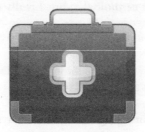

A well-respected surgeon was relaxing on his sofa one evening just after arriving home from work. As he was tuning into the evening news, the phone rang. The doctor calmly answered it and heard the familiar voice of a colleague on the other end of the line.
"We need a fourth for poker," said the friend.
"I'll be right over," whispered the doctor.
As he was putting on his coat, his wife asked,
"Is it serious?"
"Oh yes, quite serious," said the doctor gravely. "In fact, three doctors are attending already!"

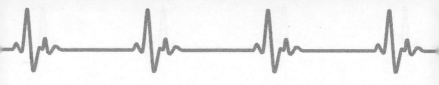

A surgeon is doing an operation. He's about to finish when, surprisingly, the patient wakes, sits up, and demands to know what's going on.

"I'm about to close," says the surgeon.

The patient grabs the surgeon's hand and says,

"I'm not going to let you do that. I'll close my own incision."

The surgeon hands him the needle and thread and says,

"OK, suture self."

During the operation the absent-minded surgeon left a sponge in the patient. She was fine – but soon found she got very thirsty.

"What's the most important thing you've learned since becoming a surgeon?"

"Take a deep breath, keep my head down, arms up and hit straight through the ball."

Before going in for surgery I thought it would be funny if I posted a cheeky note on my chest telling the surgeon to be careful. After the surgery I found another note on my body.

"I seem to have mislaid my mobile phone. Please let me know if it appears!"

A friend of mine had bone marrow cancer in his left leg and his oncologist recommended amputating the leg. After getting a second opinion that confirmed the diagnosis, my friend agreed to surgery.

When he woke up, he discovered they'd taken the wrong leg. Worse still, he still has to undergo the original amputation.

After the second surgery, my friend decided to claim from the hospital. While he claimed negligence they defended themselves by saying it was reasonable occupational error. So in the end he decided to go to court and sue the health trust. It was a futile case – he could only afford a local solicitor while the Trust brought out the expensive hot-shot lawyers. The judge ruled he didn't have a leg to stand on.

> *What kind of bandage do people wear after heart surgery?*
>
> *Ticker tape.*

I had my appendix removed. There was nothing wrong with it, I just did it as a warning to the other organs in my body to shape up or they're out of there.

Another 10 Things You Don't Want to Hear During Surgery

🚑 Go and whisper in his ear to "Move away from the light".

🚑 Hey, if you pull on this it makes a funny noise.

🚑 I guess there's a first time for everything.

🚑 Oops! Has anyone seen my watch?

🚑 Anyone seen that pink bit – it's long, thin and squelchy?

🚑 Now for an old trick I learned in my days at the veterinary college.

🚑 Jeez! Take a picture. This is truly a freak of nature.

🚑 If I can just remember how they did this on Holby last week.

🚑 I don't know what it is, but hurry up and pack it in ice.

🚑 Just pick off the fluff. It'll be ok; the floor was cleaned this morning.

Jake and Ted were out cutting wood, and Ted cut his arm off. Jake wrapped the arm in a plastic bag and took it and Ted to a surgeon. The surgeon said,

"You're in luck! I'm an expert at re-attaching limbs! Leave it with me and come back in four hours."

So Jake came back in four hours and the surgeon said,

"I finished the operation much quicker than I expected. Ted is down at the local pub."

Jake went to the pub and was amazed to see Ted throwing darts. A few weeks later, Jake and Ted were out in the woods again, and Ted somehow managed to cut his leg off. Jake put the leg in a plastic bag and took it and Ted back to the surgeon. The surgeon said,

"Legs are a little tougher – leave it with me and come back in six hours."

Jake returned in six hours and the surgeon said,

"I finished early again – Ted's down at the sports centre."

Jake went to the sports centre and there was Ted, playing up front in a football match.

A few weeks later, Ted had a terrible accident and cut his head off. Jake put the head in a plastic bag and took it and the rest of Ted to the surgeon. The surgeon said,

"Gee, heads are really tough. You best come back in twelve hours."

So Jake returned in twelve hours and the surgeon said,

"I'm sorry, Ted died." Jake said, "I understand – heads must be the most difficult of all." The surgeon said, "Oh, no! The surgery would have been fine! Ted suffocated in that plastic bag!"

I was a young junior doctor called upon to assist in surgery on a new-born child. He was his mother's pride and joy but unfortunately the baby had been born with no eyelids. With gauze on his eyes to keep them moist, the surgeon decided to try a new skin graft therapy utilizing the foreskin to shape eyelids and tendons from the fingers to allow the child to blink.

Years later I was doing my rounds as a senior registrar when I came across the very same boy – now a young man just leaving university. He was in hospital for a football injury, a broken leg I recall but apart from that he was, to the layman anyway, completely normal. I, however, couldn't help noticing he was still a little cock-eyed.

"Apparently I need foot surgery. But I would prefer the doctor to use his hands!"

What's the Story, Doc?

A young doctor moved out to a small community to replace the aging doctor there. The older doctor suggested that the younger doctor accompany him as he made his house calls so that the people of the community could become accustomed to him.

At the first house they visited, the younger doctor listened intently as the older doctor and an older lady discussed the weather, their grandchildren and the latest church bulletin. After some time, the older doctor asked his patient how she had been feeling. "I've been a little sick to my stomach," she replied. "Well," said the older physician, "you've probably been over doing it a bit with the fresh fruit. Why don't you cut back on the amount of fresh fruit you eat and see if that helps?"

As they left the house, the younger doctor asked how the older doctor had reached his diagnosis so quickly. "You didn't even examine that woman," the younger doctor stated. "I didn't have to," the elder physician explained. "You noticed that I dropped my stethoscope on the floor in there. Well when I bent over to pick it up, I looked around and noticed a half dozen banana peels in the trash can. That is probably what has been making her ill."

"That's pretty sneaky," commented the younger doctor. "Do you mind if I try it at the next house?" "I don't suppose it could hurt anything," the elder physician replied. At the next house, the two doctors visited with an elderly widow. They spent several minutes discussing the weather and grandchildren and the latest church bulletin. After several minutes, the younger doctor asked the widow how she had been feeling lately. "I've felt terribly run down lately," the widow replied. "I just don't have as much energy as I used to." "You've probably been doing too much work for the church," the younger doctor suggested without even examining his patient. "Perhaps you should ease up a bit and see if that helps." As they left, the elder physician said, "Your diagnosis is probably right, but do you mind telling me how you came to that conclusion?" "Sure," replied the younger doctor. "Just like you, I dropped my stethoscope on the floor. When I bent down to pick it up, I looked around and there was the preacher hiding under the bed!"

> *I read in the paper today that after a research appeal the NHS have been inundated with anonymous stool samples.*
> *And that made me think – Who gives a sh**?*

A handsome young lad went into the hospital for some minor surgery and the day after the procedure, a friend stopped by to see how the guy was doing. The friend was amazed at the number of nurses who entered the room in short intervals with refreshments, offers to fluff his pillows, make the bed, give back rubs, etc.

"Why all the attention ?" the friend asked. "You look fine to me."

"I know!" grinned the patient. "But the nurses seem to have changed their attitude when they heard that my circumcision required twenty-seven stitches."

John was successful in his career, but as he got older he was increasingly hampered at work by terrible headaches. When his personal hygiene and love life started to suffer, he sought medical help. After being referred from one specialist to another, he finally came across a doctor who solved the problem.

"The good news is I can cure your headaches. The bad news is that it will require castration. You have a rare condition which causes your testicles to press up against the base of your spine. The pressure creates one hell of a headache. The only way to relieve the pressure is to remove the testicles."

John was shocked and depressed. He wondered if he had anything to live for. He couldn't concentrate long enough to answer, but decided he had no choice but to go under the knife.

When he left the hospital, his mind was clear for the first time since he could remember, but he felt like he was missing an important part of himself.

As he walked down the street, he realized he felt like a different person. He could make a new beginning and live a new life. In fact, he had no choice. He walked past a men's clothing store and thought, "That's what I need: a new suit."

He entered the shop and told the salesman, "I'd like a new suit." The salesman eyed him briefly and said, "Let's see... size 44 long." John laughed. "That's right! How did you know?" The salesman smiled. "It's my job." John tried on the suit. It fit perfectly.

As he admired himself in the mirror, the salesman asked, "How about a new shirt?" John thought for a moment, and then said, "Sure." The salesman eyed him and said, "Let's see... 34 sleeve, 16½ neck". John was surprised, "That's right, how come you knew?"

"It's my job."

John tried on the shirt, and it fit perfectly.

As he adjusted the collar in the mirror, the salesman asked, "How about some new shoes?" John was on a roll. "Sure." The salesman eyed John's feet and said, "Let's see... 9½ ?" John was incredulous. "Let me guess. It's your job?"

"Right."

John tried on the shoes and they fit perfectly.

John walked comfortably around the shop and the salesman asked, "How about a new hat?" Without hesitating, John said, "Sure." The salesman eyed John's head and said, "Let's see... 7 and 5/8". John, more amazed than ever, didn't say anything this time. The hat fit perfectly.

John was feeling like a million dollars when the salesman asked, "How about some new underwear?" John hesitated, remembering his new circumstance and said, "OK." The salesman stepped back, eyed John's waist and said, "Let's see... size 36."

John laughed. "You're finally got one wrong, but not by much. I've worn size 34 since I was 18 years old." The salesman frowned and shook his head.

"No, no.no. You can't wear a size 34. It would press your testicles up against the base of your spine and give you one hell of a headache."

The NHS

*We had our first child on the NHS. It was absolutely terrible.
We had to wait nine months.*

I sat down for breakfast this morning about to eat my cereal.
I glanced down and took exception to the dish I had my
cornflakes in. So I swapped it for a saucer. However, I still
didn't like that so I exchanged it for a dish. This still didn't
appeal to me, so I then used a big cup. This also didn't look
right so I gave up. I rang NHS Direct and they drew my
attention to a complaint called 'Irritable Bowl Syndrome'.

Doctors just found a gene for shyness. They would have
found it earlier, but it was hiding behind a couple of other
genes.

If the Government wants to shorten NHS waiting lists, why
don't they just use a smaller font?

Time can heal all wounds. That explains why NHS waiting
lists are so long.

Say what you like about the NHS but it has its advantages.
I usually go private but I've recently had a few money
problems. I've had trouble being able to urinate so I
decided to get my problem looked at free of charge on the
NHS. I didn't spend a penny.

My 92 year old grandmother was complaining that she been on the NHS waiting list for an operation for over a year. I agreed it was really not acceptable, especially for a woman of her age. But as I said to her, "Gran, could you not just live without bigger boobs?"

A man enters hospital for treatment in one of the government's flagship hospitals. He finds himself greeted by an NHS administrator. The smartly dressed man says "Welcome to a new NHS where we recognize your choices are important." He offers the new patient a seat and gets out a glossy brochure. "First of all," he continues. "we can offer you a room with an ocean view or a forest view." The man is pretty impressed. "That's great." he says. "I'll take the ocean view, thanks."
"No problem," says the administrator, picking up a phone. "I'll get them to switch the posters right away."

> *I heard on the news tonight that alcohol was costing the NHS £2.6 billion a year. They really should think about cutting down a little.*

Found on NHS medical records (Part One)

🚑 By the time he was admitted, his rapid heart had stopped, and he was feeling better.

🚑 Patient has chest pain if she lies on her left side for over a year.

🚑 On the second day the knee was better and on the third day it had completely disappeared.

🚑 She has had no rigors or shaking chills, but her husband states she was very hot in bed last night.

🚑 The patient has been depressed ever since she began seeing me in 1983.

🚑 Patient was released to outpatient department without dressing.

🚑 I have suggested that he loosen his pants before standing, and then, when he stands with the help of his wife, they should fall to the floor.

🚑 The patient is tearful and crying constantly. She also appears to be depressed.

🚑 Discharge status: Alive but without permission.

🚑 The patient will need disposition, and therefore we will get the doctor to dispose of him.

🚑 Healthy appearing decrepit 69 year-old male, mentally alert but forgetful.

The patient refused an autopsy.

The patient has no past history of suicides.

The patient expired on the floor uneventfully.

Patient has left his white blood cells at another hospital.

The patient's past medical history has been remarkably insignificant with only a 40 pound weight gain in the past three days.

She slipped on the ice and apparently her legs went in separate directions in early December.

The patient experienced sudden onset of severe shortness of breath with a picture of acute pulmonary oedema at home while having sex which gradually deteriorated in the emergency room.

The patient had waffles for breakfast and anorexia for lunch.

Between you and me, we ought to be able to get this lady pregnant.

The patient was in his usual state of good health until his aircraft ran out of fuel and crashed.

Since she can't get pregnant with her husband, I thought you would like to work her up.

She is numb from her toes down.

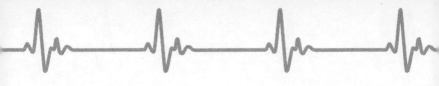

🚑 While in the ER, she was examined, X-rated and sent home.

🚑 Occasional, constant, infrequent headaches.

🚑 Patient was alert and unresponsive.

🚑 When she fainted, her eyes rolled around the room.

The latest round of cuts to the National Health Service didn't go down well with The British Medical Association...

The **Allergists** voted to scratch the proposal, and the **Dermatologists** advised not to make any rash moves.

The **Gastroenterologist**s had a sort of a gut feeling about it, but the **Neurologists** thought the Government had a lot of nerve.

The **Obstetricians** felt they were all labouring under a misconception while the **Ophthalmologists** considered the idea short-sighted.

The **Psychiatrists** thought the whole idea was madness, while the **Radiologists** could see right through it.

The **Pharmacologists** thought it was a bitter pill to swallow; the **Proctologists** thought it a pain in the arse; the **Urologists** were pissed off at the whole idea and the **Pathologists** yelled, "Over my dead body!"

10 unexpected categories of 2011 NHS admissions

Crocodile or Alligator bites (2)
Scorpion bites (6)
People aged over 75 falling out of a tree (12)
Volcanic eruptions victims (15)
Earthquake victims (5)
Foreign object left in body after surgery (156)
Prolonged stay in weightless environment (4)
Caught in Avalanche (10)
Drowning and submersion while in bath tub (43)
Hardboiled egg in orifice (1)

> *My wife had our baby last night.*
>
> *12 pounds...*
>
> *These NHS car parks are daylight robbery!*

According to a new NHS directive a Patient is not 'dead'...
He is 'electroencephalographically-challenged'.

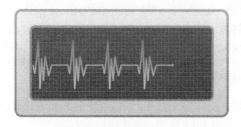

Found on NHS medical records (Part Two)

- The lab test indicated abnormal lover function.

- The baby was delivered, the cord clamped and cut, and handed to the paediatrician, who breathed and cried immediately.

- Exam of genitalia reveals that he is circus sized.

- She stated that she had been constipated for most of her life until 1989 when she got a divorce.

- The patient lives at home with his mother, father, and pet turtle, who is presently enrolled in day care three times a week.

- Both breasts are equal and reactive to light and accommodation.

- Exam of genitalia was completely negative except for the right foot.

- The patient was to have a bowel resection. However, he took a job as stockbroker instead.

- The patient is a 79-year-old widow who no longer lives with her husband.

- Many years ago the patient had frostbite of the right shoe.

- The patient left the hospital feeling much better except for her original complaints.

A policeman stops a drink driver and asks him to take a breath test.

The driver pulls out a NHS card which reads,
This man is asthmatic please don't take his breath.

The policeman then asks him to take a blood test. The man pulls out another NHS card.
This man is anaemic please don't take his blood.

The policeman starts to lose his patience and asks the man to take a urine test.

The driver pulls out a third card:
This man is a Spurs supporter, please don't take the piss!

I feel sorry for that amputee guy who, having lost his right foot, was given 2 left feet by mistake.
He's been trying for months to claim from the NHS, but feels he is going round in circles.

The Boat Race

There was once a boat race organized in which a British NHS team took on a Japanese health team. Both teams took the race really seriously, picked their best athletes and trained hard. The NHS team believed they had a great chance of victory but come the race day the Japanese won by 20 lengths.

The NHS team were devastated by the result and morale sagged. So senior management organized a re-match a year later – vowing that in the meantime the reason for the crushing defeat had to be found.

A working party was set up to investigate the problem and recommend appropriate action. After careful consideration, they concluded that the Japanese team had eight people rowing and one person steering, whereas the NHS. team had eight people steering and one person rowing.

Senior Management immediately hired a consultancy company to do a study on the team's structure. Millions of pounds and several months later they concluded that 'too many people were steering and not enough rowing'.

To prevent losing to the Japanese next year, the team structure was changed to three Assistant Steering Managers, three Steering Managers, one Executive Steering Manager and a Director of Steering Services. A performance and appraisal system was set up to give the person rowing the boat more incentive to work harder.

The next year the Japanese won by 40 lengths.

Following this, the NHS. laid off the rower for poor performance, sold off all the paddles, cancelled all capital investment for new equipment, and halted development of a new boat. The money saved was used to fund bigger bonuses for Senior Management.

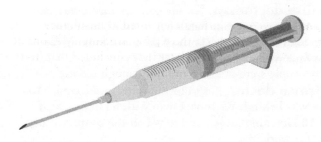

> *The hospital made a real mess of my brain surgery.*
>
> *I've half a mind to sue.*

A Japanese doctor says, "Medicine in our country is so advanced that we can take a kidney out of one man, put it in another, and have him out looking for work in six weeks."

A German doctor says, "That is nothing. We can take a lung out of one person, put it in another, and have him out looking for work in four weeks."

A Swedish doctor says, "In my country medicine is so advanced that we can take half a heart out of one person, put it in another, and have both of them out looking for work in four weeks."

The British doctor, not to be outdone, interjected, "You guys are way behind. We took a man with no brains, sent him to 10 Downing Street, and now half the country is out looking for work."

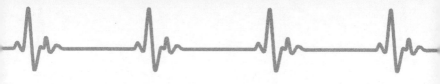

A new medical facility with several different specialists opened in a trendy part of the city. Wanting to be different and creative, the administration decided that each doctor's office door would, in some way, be representative of his practice.
So, when construction was complete...
the opthalmic consultant's door had a peep hole,
the orthopaedist's door had a broken hinge,
the psychiatrist's door was painted all kinds of crazy colours,
and the gynaecologist's door was left open... just a crack.

Britain's Health Minister has denied that there are plans to rebrand the NHS as 'The Sick Factor' where patients looking for treatment will have to convince a panel of doctors they are sick enough to get a place in hospital.

> *WARNING if you get an email from the government warning you of the dangers of swine flu from tinned pork.*
> *DONT OPEN IT. ITS JUST SPAM.*

Honestly, the state of the NHS these days. A new report claims 4 out of 5 doctors recommend another doctor.

> *I think the NHS cutbacks have gone too far...*
> *I didn't even get a sticker at the dentist today.*

Calling older patients "dearie" or "love" is set to be ruled out as offensive by new guidelines from the Nursing and Midwifery Council. However, it doesn't say anything about calling them "coffin dodging, piss-stained old gits".

> *The NHS are apparently now paying sixty quid*
> *for sperm donations... that makes the old towel*
> *under my bed worth a few grand.*

> *I received a letter from my consultant at the sexual health clinic to tell me that I'm the most important man he's ever treated. I've never been treated so well by the NHS, and if the people at my local dyslexia support centre are half as nice, I'll be delighted.*

This NHS Direct is brilliant, just like going to the doctors. I logged in and inputted all my symptoms and it gave me a diagnosis and printed out what tablets to take... in a font I couldn't read.

> *The NHS really is rubbish. On their report they wrote that I had type P blood, but it was a Type-O.*

I for one was very disappointed with NHS Direct. When my daughter cut her arm I rang them straight away and they told me to put a light dressing on it. I made lovely vinaigrette, but she screamed the place down and it really didn't help at all.

Homeopathy

Homeopathy. Nothing works as well.

A motto for reluctant homeopathic pharmacists:
"We who are about to sigh dilute thee."

How many homeopaths does it take to change a light bulb?
None. You can't just change the bulb you need to change the whole house.

I invented the homoeopathic Viagra.
It does work, but you need to rub it on really well.

Did you hear about the suicidal homeopath?
He took a massive underdose...

Many people swear by homeopathy. Even our own Prince of Wales has claimed the alternative treatments have some merit. Many of my friends – otherwise educated, cultured people – say it can help them recover from a cold in just seven days. They are right of course; left alone it would probably take a whole week.

What do you call alternative medicine that has been scientifically proven to work?
Medicine.

Hear about the homeopathic doctor who wanted to get completely drunk.
He went to his local and ordered half a shot of whisky and ten gallons of water.

Did you hear about the American podiatrist and the English chiropodist?
They were arch rivals.

An anthropologist was on a lecture tour in the UK recounting his encounters with a little-contacted African tribe. While telling of his friendship with a local witch doctor, he explained how we should be cautious about being too sceptical of tribal medicines.

"For instance," he said, "at one time I was in a really bad way. I tried to relay my symptoms to the witch doctor but with our language differences it was very difficult."

To his audience's great delight, the academic then began by repeating the mime he had performed – crouching down, screwing up his eyes and straining. Like the tribesman before them, the audience guessed the problem immediately – constipation!

"So," continued the lecturer. "he beckoned me to follow and led me into the jungle to a particular fern. He gathered up some leaves and returned to the camp and boiled them up. And, do you know Ladies and Gentlemen; they cleared me out like nothing I've ever known. Yep. Let me tell you, with fronds like these, who needs enemas!"

There were two doctors in a bar, spending the evening moaning about the current state of the NHS, government interference, hospital managers, crap IT, abusive patients, litigious patients, rotas, paperwork, overwork, lack of time with patients who need it etc, etc.

The first says, "I don't know. I'm so peed off with it all I feel like jacking it in and getting into alternative medicine. I have been considering becoming a chiropractor."

"A chiroquacktor?" laughs the second doctor. "You're joking aren't you? You'd really quit being a respected doctor for some jumped-up pseudo medical occupation?"

"Yep, I'm serious," says the first. "I've thought it through. I can keep my "Dr" title and a have brass plaque on the front door of my own private practice. I have a string of patients with mainly back problems and a few sporting injuries. I'll crack their bones, charge them through the nose, and they won't know if it's working or not. I can set my own practice hours. Go home at regular times. Play plenty of golf. It will be fantastic."

"Admittedly that all sounds good," says his understanding friend, "but you'll have to go on a long training course and get a new degree. It could take years."

"That's true," replies the other. "Really I just want to get through all that and start cracking bones."

"Mmmm," says doctor number two. "Maybe I can help you there". "As a renowned brain surgeon I have been trialling a new procedure. It's experimental, but I am having a few successes. If you were happy to be my guinea pig I could perform an operation will basically instantly transform you from a doctor into a chiropractor."

"Is that possible?" asks the first.

"Yes, in layman's terms, simplifying things somewhat, what we do is remove half your brain."

Looking rather alarmed, the first says, "Good grief! That sounds serious. I'm not sure I could go through with that!"

"Well, it's not so bad," reassures the brain surgeon. "We are very particular about which parts of the brain we remove. We shall pick out all those bits that got stuffed full of anatomy and physiology at medical school. Obviously we shall leave some remnants of basic medical knowledge there and let you believe that you have a fully equivalent medical training in such areas. Out will go all that stuff on pharmacology, biochemistry, anaesthesiology, surgery and psychiatry along with any basic understanding of science.

"Wow! Fantastic!" says the first.

"I can fit you in this afternoon, if that's OK?" says the second.

The doctor went ahead with the operation but unfortunately the procedure went horribly wrong. As the first doctor starts coming round from the anaesthetic, the surgeon is waiting to break the bad news. "I'm afraid, the operation did not go as planned," he says.

"What do you mean?"

"Due to a mix up with some paperwork, we accidentally removed your whole brain. We tried our best, but were unable to restore those areas you will need to become a chiropractor. I am afraid you have no brain."

"Never mind." says the surprisingly chirpy and optimistic patient. "I think I will just become a homeopath."

Cosmetic Surgery

When it comes to cosmetic surgery, a lot of people turn their noses up.

> *My wife said she fancied some plastic surgery. So I cut up all her credit cards.*

A cosmetic surgeon recently set up surgery in my staid little town.
He raised a few eyebrows.

Remember to be specific in plastic surgery requests. My wife just came back from getting a boob job with 'silly cone implants.'

I am so unlucky. I lent my friend £3,000 for plastic surgery and now I don't know what he looks like.

My wife went to have a face-lift last week, but when they saw what was under it they dropped it again.

One plastic surgeon said to another: "my daughter gets her good looks from me."

A woman in the bar says that she wants to have plastic surgery to enlarge her breasts. Her husband tells her, "Hey, you don't need surgery to do that. I know how to do it without surgery."

The lady asks, "How do I do it without surgery?" He replies, "Just rub toilet paper between them."

"How on earth will that make them bigger?" she demands. "I don't know," he says as he eases away. "But it worked for your arse."

My wife had a non-surgical face lift. She was quite pleased with it but to be honest she should have paid out for a proper operation. I could see some of the sellotape at the sides.

My wife's breast augmentation went tits up.

> *My wife's saving up for a second boob job. Well, I've got to be honest, she does look ridiculous with one big and one small one.*

As a plastic surgeon, women often ask my advice on breast enlargement. I find I can usually give them a couple of pointers.

Osteopaths and Chiropractors

What's the difference between a rhinoceros and an orthopaedic surgeon?
One's thick-skinned, small-brained and charges a lot for no very good reason... the other's a rhinoceros.

> *Osteoporosis*
> *...it's not what is cracked up to be.*

Why aren't there any osteopaths in Egypt?
Because they're all Cairo-practors!

Did you hear about the man who had been subscribing to Osteopathy Magazine for over 20 years?
He had plenty of back issues.

Did you hear the one about the psychiatric chiropractor?
He specializes in attitude adjustments!

In a long line of people waiting for a bank clerk, one guy suddenly started massaging the back of the person in front of him. Surprised, the man in front turned and snarled, "Just what the hell you are doing?"
"Well," said the guy, "You see, I'm a chiropractor and I could see that you were tense, so I had to massage your back. Sometimes I just can't help practising my art!"
"That's the stupidest thing I've ever heard!" the guy replied. "I'm a lawyer. Do you see me screwing the guy in front of me?"

Q: What kind of music do chiropractors listen to?
A: Hip-Pop!

Chiropractor: Good morning, Ms Jones. If you'll lie down on the table, we can begin your adjustment.
Patient: Thanks, Doctor. And I have to thank you for being so personable about your work. I've heard that the way to make money as a chiropractor is to run as many people through your office as you can each day, assembly-line style, without giving...
Chiropractor (interrupting): Well, if that's all, then I will see you again in a week.

Santa's sledge broke down on Christmas Eve. He flagged down a passing motorist and asked, "Can you help me fix my sledge?"
"Sorry," the motorist replied. "I'm afraid I'm not a mechanic – I'm a podiatrist."
"Well," said Santa, "can you give me a toe?"

Podiatrists. They've gained a real foothold in the medical profession.

> *What kind of jokes does a podiatrist like?*
> *Corny jokes.*

"I stand corrected," said the man in the orthopaedic shoes.

At the Vets

Eric took his Saint Bernard to the vet.
"Doctor," he said sadly, "I'm afraid I'm going to
have to ask you to cut off my dog's tail."
The vet stepped back,
"Eric, why should I do such a terrible thing?"
"Because my mother-in-law's arriving tomorrow,
and I don't want anything to make her think
she's welcome."

A woman calls a vet and says she hasn't been able to sleep because her dog snores too loudly. The vet tells her to tie a ribbon around his balls and he will shut up. The woman goes to her bedroom and sees her dog lying on the floor snoring. She gets a red ribbon and ties it around his balls. The dog stops snoring. The woman goes to sleep.

After a while, her husband comes home drunk. He lies in bed and falls fast asleep. He starts to snore loudly so the woman gets a blue ribbon and ties it around his balls. The next morning the woman gets up and goes to work. The man wakes up and sees the blue ribbon on his balls. Then he looks down at the dog and sees the red ribbon around his balls. The guy says to the dog, "I don't know what we did last night, but we got first and second place!'"

A man took his cross-eyed dog to the vet and asked, "Is there anything you can do for him?"

The vet picked the dog up and peered into his eyes. "I'm going to have to put him down," the vet said finally.

"Just because he's cross-eyed?" asked the owner.

"No, because he's heavy," said the vet.

A woman takes her hamster to the vets. Her precious pet is clearly dead but the woman is distraught so the vet looks at its eyes, and gets his stethoscope out to have a listen to its heart before gently explaining that the hamster is deceased. The woman refuses to accept it. "Are you sure," she cries. "Are there no more checks you can do?"

"There is one more definitive procedure we can go through but it is costly," suggests the vet. He then goes into the next room and returns with a lovely chocolate Labrador. The dog puts its front paws on the table and sniffs the hamster up and down before looking at the vet with its big brown eyes and shaking its head. The vet then takes the dog out and returns with a big, fluffy ginger cat which he places on the table. It then proceeds to lick the hamster up and down before turning to look at the vet and shake its head sadly.

"Well that confirms it,"announces the vet. "I'm really sorry. There is nothing more we can do for your hamster. It is deceased. And I'm afraid the bill comes to £350."

"How come it cost so much?" asks the woman, still confused and upset.

"Well," he says, "it is £200 for the lab tests and £150 for the cat scan."

A man buys several sheep, hoping to breed them for wool. After several weeks, he notices that none of the sheep are getting pregnant, and calls a vet for help. The vet tells him that he should try artificial insemination.

The guy doesn't have the slightest idea what this means but not wanting to display his ignorance, only asks the vet how he will know when the sheep are pregnant. The vet tells him that they will stop standing around and will lie down and wallow in the grass. The man hangs up and gives it some thought. He comes to the conclusion that artificial insemination means he has to impregnate the sheep. So he loads the sheep into his truck, drives them out into the woods, has sex with them all, brings them back, and goes to bed.

The next morning he wakes to find the sheep still just standing around. One more try, he tells himself, and proceeds to load them up and drive them out to the woods. He spends all day shagging the sheep and upon returning home, falls listlessly into bed.

The next morning, he wakes and looks out at the sheep. Seeing that they are all still standing around, he concludes that the first try didn't take, and loads them in the truck again. He drives them out to the woods, bangs each sheep twice for good measure, brings them back, and goes to bed.

The next morning, he cannot even raise himself from the bed to look at the sheep. He asks his wife to look out and tell him if the sheep are lying in the grass.
"No," she says, "they're all in the truck and one of them is honking the horn."

A veterinarian surgeon had had a hell of a day, but when he got home from tending to all the sick animals his wife was waiting with a long cool drink and a romantic candle-lit dinner, after which they had a few more drinks and went happily to bed.

At about 2:00 in the morning, the phone rang. "Is this the vet?" asked an elderly lady's voice.

"Yes, it is," replied the vet, "is this an emergency?"

"Well, sort of," said the elderly lady, "there's a whole bunch of cats on the roof outside making a terrible noise mating and I can't get to sleep. What can I do about it?"

There was a sharp intake of breath from the vet, who then patiently replied:

"Open the window and tell them they're wanted on the phone."

"Really?" said the elderly lady, "Will that will that stop them?"

"Should do," said the vet, "IT STOPPED ME."

Dr Jones had felt terrible all day long. No matter how much he tried to forget about it, he couldn't. The guilt and sense of betrayal was overwhelming. But every once in a while, he'd hear a soothing voice trying to reassure him: "David. Don't worry about it. You aren't the first doctor to sleep with one of his patients and you won't be the last." But invariably another voice would bring him back to reality. "David. They weren't veterinarians."

Another Trip to the Hospital

Two men are chatting in their hospital beds:
"What are you in for?" asked the first.
"Camera down the throat" the other replied.
"Oh endoscopy?" the first man asked.
"Yes" he said "Checking for stomach cancer. What about you?"
"Camera up the arse" he said.
"Oh colonoscopy, checking for bowel cancer?" quizzed the second man.
"No, my neighbour was sunbathing and my wife caught me taking a photo."

> *Why did the proctologist use two fingers?*
>
> *In case the patient wanted a second opinion.*

Overheard in the hospital:

"Don't worry, the doctor has seen an operation exactly like yours on TV."

The colder the X-ray table the more of your body is required on it.

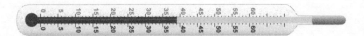

A man wakes up in the hospital bandaged from head to foot. The doctor comes in and says, "Ah, I see you've regained consciousness. Now you probably won't remember, but you were in a huge pile-up on the motorway. You're going to be okay, you'll walk and talk again, but your penis was severed in the accident and we couldn't find it."

The man groans, but the doctor goes on, "Fortunately we now have the technology to build a new penis. They look and they work great – you won't be able to tell the difference. At this, the man perks up a little.

The doc continues, "However, they don't come cheap. The cost is roughly a thousand pound an inch. So you will have to decide how many inches you want. I understand that you have been married for over thirty years and this is something you should discuss with your wife. If you had a five-incher before and get a nine-incher now, it might come as bit of a shock. Whereas if you had a nine-incher before and you decide to only invest in a five-incher now, she might be somewhat disappointed. It's important that she plays a role in helping you make a decision."

With this, the man agrees to talk it over with his wife.

The doctor comes back the next day, "So, have you spoken with your wife?"

"Yes, I have," says the man.

"And has she helped you make a decision?"

"Yes," says the man.

"What is your decision?" asks the doctor.

"We're getting granite countertops."

A man was just waking up from anaesthesia after surgery, and his wife was sitting by his side.
His eyes fluttered open and he said: "You're beautiful!" and then he fell asleep again.
His wife had never heard him say that so she stayed by his side.
A couple of minutes later his eyes fluttered open and he said: "You're really cute, you know?"
Well, the wife was disappointed because this time instead of "beautiful" he'd said "cute."
She said: "Hey last time you said I was 'beautiful', what's happened?"
He replied: "The drugs are wearing off!"

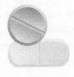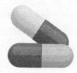

While I was working as a receptionist for an eye surgeon, a very angry woman stormed up to my desk. "Someone swapped my wig while I was having surgery yesterday," she complained.
The doctor came out and tried to calm her down. "I assure you that no one on my staff would have done such a thing," he said. "Why do you think it was taken here?"
"After the operation, I noticed the wig I was wearing was cheap-looking and ugly."
"I think," explained the surgeon gently, "that means your cataract operation was a success."

A man and a woman were waiting at the hospital donation unit.

Man: "What are you doing here today?"

Woman: "Oh, I'm here to donate some blood. They're going to give me £5 for it."

Man: "Hmm, that's interesting. I'm here to donate sperm, myself. But they pay me £60."

The woman looked thoughtful for a moment and they chatted some more before going their separate ways.

Several months later, the man and woman meet again in the donation unit.

Man: "Oh, hi there! Here to donate blood again?"

Woman: [shaking her head with mouth closed] "Unh unh."

> *Doesn't time fly -*
> *when you're in a coma!*

A man needing a heart transplant is told by his doctor that the only heart available is that of a sheep. The man finally agrees and the doctor transplants the sheep heart into the man. A few days after the operation, the man comes in for a check up. The doctor asks him "How are you feeling?" The man replies "Not BAAAAD!"

David Cameron is being shown around an Edinburgh hospital. Towards the end of his visit, he is shown into a ward with a number of people with no obvious signs of injury. He goes to greet the first patient and the chap replies:

"Fair fa' your honest sonsie face, Great chieftain e' the puddin' race! Aboon them a' ye tak your place, Painch, tripe, or thairm: Weel are ye wordy o' a grace as lang 's my arm."

David, a little confused, pulls that supercilious smile he has and moves on to the next patient and greets him. The next bed-ridden chap replies: "Some hae meat, and canna eat, And some wad eat that want it, But we hae meat and we can eat, And sae the Lord be thank it."

Cameron, now even more puzzled, says "Hmmm... Good man." And then moves somewhat cautiously on to the next patient and says, "Hello, how are you?"

The third immediately starts prattling on: "Wee sleekit, cow'rin, tim'rous beastie, O, what a panic's in thy breastie! Thou need na start awa sae hasty, Wi bickering brattle! I wad be laith to rin an chase thee, Wi murdering pattle!"

Cameron raises his eyebrows and turns to the doctor accompanying him, asking: "What sort of ward is this, some kind of mental ward?"

"No," replies the doctor, "It's the Serious Burns unit."

> *A man ended up in a hospital today, covered in wood and hay, with a toy horse lodged in his arse. The doctors have described his condition as stable.*

Hospital regulations require a wheelchair for patients being discharged. However, a student nurse found one elderly gentleman already dressed and sitting on the bed with a suitcase at his feet, who insisted he didn't need her help to leave the hospital.

After a chat about rules being rules, he reluctantly let her wheel him to the elevator.

On the way down she asked him if his wife was meeting him.

"I don't know," he said. "She's still upstairs in the bathroom changing out of her hospital gown."

The doctor told a woman that her husband had died of a massive myocardial infarct. Not more than five minutes later, he heard her telling the rest of the family that he had died of a "massive internal fart."

> *Our local ice cream man was brought into A&E covered in hundreds and thousands.*
>
> *Police say that he had tried to top himself.*

Doctor - "Okay, Mrs A, let's have a look at your results."
Patient - "My name isn't Mrs A."
Doctor - "Right, I have some bad news then.
  It appears you have MRSA."

A mate of mine had severe back problems and went in for that new operation last month where they inject mercury into the base of the spine. It was pretty painful but he says it seems to be helping. The only drawback so far is that he is 5ft 1 on a cold day and 6ft 4 when the sun is out.

> *My son's developed orange and white stripes on his body.*
>
> *Doctors have put him on a course of Nemotherapy.*

"I'm not going back to that physiotherapy department at the hospital."
"Why not?"
"It was that masseur. He just rubbed me up the wrong way."

After recovering from a recent car accident a man was referred to a physiotherapist.
"How flexible are you?" asked the physio.
"Well, I'm pretty flexible," replied the patient. "But I can't do Thursdays!"

Q: What's the worst part about getting a lung transplant?

A: The first couple of times you cough, it's not your phlegm.

A radiologist was conducting a radiographic examination of a woman's abdomen. Finding that her clothing was causing some interference with his monitor screen, he called out, "Would you pull down your knickers, please?"

The patient did nothing, so he was forced to repeat the request. This time he heard her say, "Oh, I'm so sorry, doctor. I thought you were talking to the nurse."

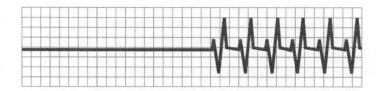

A woman takes her first child to the doctors for her immunizations. The nurse consults her records and notices the child's name is Urine. "That's a very unusual name" she comments politely, "is it a family name?"

The woman explains that Urine was very sick after she was born and had to stay in intensive care for several weeks. Distressed, the mother had not yet chosen a name for her daughter, but the nurses promised they would pray for her.

A couple of days later, the mother returns from the bathroom to find a note written on her daughter's incubator that read 'Please Save Urine'. The mother was overcome by their touching support and decided to keep the name the nurses had clearly chosen for her daughter.

In a hospital, a man had made several attempts to get into the
men's toilet, but it had always been occupied. He was now
getting a little desperate. A nurse noticed his predicament.
"Sir," she said "You may use the ladies' room if you promise
not to touch any of the buttons on the wall."
He did what he needed to, and as he sat there he noticed
the buttons he had promised not to touch. Each button was
identified by letters: WW, WA, PP, and a red one labelled ATR.
Who would know if he touched them? He thought. He couldn't
resist. He pushed the button marked WW and warm water
sprayed gently upon his bottom. What a lovely feeling, he
thought. Men's toilets don't have nice things like this. Now
intrigued, he pushed the WA button. Warm air replaced the
warm water, gently drying the underside of his bum. When
this stopped, he pushed the PP button. A large powder puff
caressed his bottom adding a fragile scent of spring flowers to
this unbelievable pleasure.
"Whoo hey!" he cried. This was more than a toilet – it's more
of a spa. When the powder puff completed its pleasure, he
couldn't wait to push the ATR button. He couldn't work out
what it meant but he had a feeling that this would be the best
experience yet.
The next thing he knew he was waking up in a hospital bed
with a nurse was staring down at him. "What happened?" he
exclaimed. The last thing I remember was pushing the ATR
button. "The button ATR is an Automatic Tampon Remover.
If you want to see your penis again you best look under your
pillow."

South African newspaper The Cape Times reported that over a period of a few months, every Friday staff would find one of their patients dead in their bed. It was always the same bed. First, it was passed off as a coincidence. Then staff began to suspect some terrible disease was killing their patients.

Then one day a nurse watched the cleaner as she came in on a Friday. The maid would enter the ward, unplug the life support system by the side of the bed, plug in her floor polisher, clean, plug the patient back in and leave – without noticing the now deceased patient lying in the bed.

When a baby toddler swallows a tiny magnet, the mother rushes him to casualty.

"He'll be fine, he'll be fine," the doctor reassures her. "The magnet should pass through his system in a day or so. In the meantime, however, I'd like to keep him in just for observation."

The mother goes home and returns the next day, "Doctor," she asks. "how's my baby doing?"

"Oh, he's fine, he's in the kitchen, it shouldn't be too long now."

"The kitchen?" says the woman. "Ahhhhhh! Poor thing must be starving, is he having his breakfast?"

"No, we stuck him on the refrigerator door and as soon as he falls off, you'll have that magnet back."

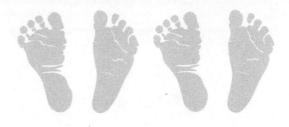

I shouldn't say my brother-in-law is tight.
He took me out for tea and biscuits last week.
Ok, so I had to give blood first...

A radiology technician took some X-rays of a trauma patient and took the results to the senior radiologist, who studied the multiple fractures of the femurs and pelvis.

"What on earth happened to this patient?" he asked in astonishment.

"He fell out of a tree," according to the report.

The radiologist wanted to know what the patient was doing up a tree.

"I'm not sure, but his paperwork states he works for Mark"s Expert Tree Pruning Service."

Gazing intently at the X-rays, the radiologist blinked and said, "Cross out 'expert'."

What is the difference between a haematologist
and a urologist?

A haematologist pricks your finger.

One day two carrots were walking down the street. They were the best of friends. Just as they started to step off the curb a car came speeding around the corner and ran one of them over.

The unharmed carrot called an ambulance and helped his friend as best he could. He was taken to the A&E department at the local hospital, and rushed away.

After many hours of agonized waiting, the doctor came out. He walked over to the distraught carrot and said

"I have good news, and I have bad news.
The good news is that your friend is going
to pull through."

"The bad news is that he's going to be a vegetable for the rest of his life".

A doctor was examining a woman who was rushed to the emergency ward. He kept her under observation and studied her charts for some time. Concerned with what he had seen, he took the woman's husband aside, and said, "I don't like how your wife looks at all."
To which the husband promptly replied, "Me neither Doc. But she's a great cook and really good with the kids!"

All in your Mind

You have made great progress," said a psychiatrist, complimenting his patient. "Progress? You call this progress," came the angry reply. "Three months ago I thought I was God – now I know I'm a nobody."

A doctor of psychology was doing his normal morning rounds when he entered the room of a patient named John. He found John sitting on the floor, pretending to saw a piece of wood. Another patient Barry was hanging from the ceiling, by his feet. The doctor asked John what he was doing. He replied, "Can't you see I'm sawing this piece of wood in half?"
And what on earth did he think Barry was up to? John replied, "Oh. He's my friend, but he's a little crazy. He thinks he's a light bulb." The doctor looks up. Barry's face is going really red. So the doctor tells John, "Listen, if he really is your friend, you should get him down from there before he hurts himself." John stops his sawing for an instant and replies: "What? And work in the dark?"

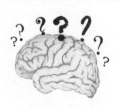

Several people were waiting for their psychiatrist in the waiting room one day.

One says to the other, "Why are you here?"

The second answers, "I'm Napoleon reincarnated. For some reason that means I have to see a doctor."

The first said, "How do you know that you were reborn as Napoleon?"

The second responds, "God told me I was."

A third person on the other side of the room stands up, points at the second, and shouts, "NO, I DID NOT!"

Bob hadn't had a good night's sleep for years. He became convinced that there were monsters under his bed and worked himself up into a terrible state every night. He'd been seeing a psychoanalyst for four years but progress had been very slow. Frustrated, he decided to try seeing a different psychoanalyst. A few weeks later, Bob bumps into his old psychoanalyst in the local supermarket. The shrink is surprised to find him looking well-rested, energetic, and cheerful.

"Doc!" Bob says, "It's really incredible! I've been cured!"

"That's great news!" the psychoanalyst says. "You seem like a different person. What happened?"

"Well I went to see another doctor," Joe began enthusiastically, "and he cured me in just ONE session!"

"One!" the psychoanalyst replied incredulously." What did he do that I couldn't?"

"Well," says Joe. "he told me to cut the legs off of my bed."

Neurotics build castles in the air.
Psychotics live in them.
Psychiatrists are the people who collect the rent.

A man bumped into an old friend in the street. "How have you been?" he enquired. "Well to be honest," came the reply, "I've been seeing a psychiatrist – I started to believe I was a Labrador." He could see his friend looked concerned so quickly added. "but I'm ok now. Just feel my nose."

Isn't it funny that when we talk to God they call it called praying, but when God talks to us, the shrink says we have delusions of grandeur!

Two psychiatrists are riding bikes.
One of them falls, and hurts himself badly, bruises and blood all over the place.
What is the other ones' response?
"Do you want to talk about it?"

A trainee psychiatrist visited a local mental institution and asked a patient, "How did you get here? What was the nature of your illness?" He got this reply...

"Well, it all started when I got married and I guess I should never have done it. I got hitched to a widow with a grown daughter who then became my stepdaughter. My daddy came to visit us; fell in love with my lovely stepdaughter, then married her. And so my stepdaughter was now my stepmother. Soon, my wife had a son who was, of course, my daddy's brother-in-law since he is the half-brother of my stepdaughter, who is now, of course, my daddy's wife.

So, as I told you, when my stepdaughter married my daddy, she was at once my stepmother! and now, since my new son is brother to my stepmother, he also became my uncle. As you know, my wife is my step-grandmother since she is my stepmother's mother. Don't forget that my stepmother is my stepdaughter. Remember, too, that I am my wife's grandson. But hold on just a few minutes more. You see, since I'm married to my step-grandmother, I am not only my wife's grandson and her hubby, but I am also my own grandfather. Now can you understand how I got put in this place?"

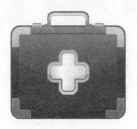

A psychiatrist was conducting a group therapy session with four young mothers and their small children.

You all have obsessions," he observed.

"To the first mother," he said, "You are obsessed with eating. You've even named your daughter Candy."

He turned to the second Mom. "Your obsession is with money. Again, it manifests itself in your child's name, Penny."

He turns to the third Mom. "Your obsession is alcohol. This too manifests itself in your child's name, Brandy."

At this point, the fourth mother gets up, takes her little boy by the hand and whispers "come on Richard, we're leaving."

My Doctor says I'm paranoid. I can't help wondering who else he's told.

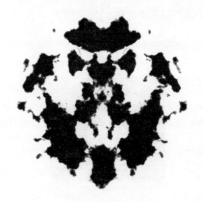

John and David were both patients in a mental hospital. One day while they were walking past the hospital swimming pool, John suddenly dived into the deep end. He sunk to the bottom and stayed there. David promptly jumped in to save him. He swam to the bottom of the pool and pulled John out. The Medical Director came to know of David's heroic act. He immediately ordered that David be discharged from the mental hospital as he considered him to be okay.

The doctor told David, "We have good news and bad news for you, David! The good news is that we are going to discharge you because you have regained your senses. Since you were able to jump in and save another patient you must be mentally stable. The bad news is that John, the patient whom you saved, hung himself in the bathroom, and died." David replied, "Doctor he didn't hang himself, I hung him there to dry."

> *My shrink thinks I'm paranoid. OK, He didn't actually say it, but I know he's thinking it.*

> *I stopped taking Prozac. I was starting to be nice to people I was deliberately ignoring.*

Hello. Welcome to the Psychiatric Hotline...

If you are anal retentive,

please hold.

If you are anxious,

just start pressing numbers at random.

If you are co-dependent,

please ask someone to press 2.

If you are delusional,

press 7 and your call will be
transferred to the Mother Ship.

If you are dyslexic,

press 9696969696969696.

If you have low self esteem,

please hang up now. All our
operators are too busy to talk to you.

If you are manic-depressive,

it doesn't matter which number
you press. No one will answer.

If you have multiple personalities,

please press 3, 4, 5, and 6.

If you have a nervous disorder,

*please fiddle with the * key until*
a representative comes on the line.

If you are obsessive-compulsive,

please press 1 repeatedly.

If you are paranoid-delusional,

> *we know who you are and what you want. Just stay on the line so we can trace the call.*

If you are phobic,

> *don't press anything.*

If you have post traumatic stress disorder,

> *slowly and carefully press 000 .*

If you are schizophrenic,

> *listen carefully and a little voice will tell you which number to press.*

If you have short term memory loss,

> *press 9. If you have short term memory loss, press 9. If you have short term memory loss, press 9.*

> *We used to take life with a grain of salt. Now it's with 5 milligrams of Prozac.*

At the psychiatrist's office a woman came in depressed.
"I feel so ugly. People won't even look me in the face.
Can you help me?"
Psychiatrist: "I think I can. Go lie face down on the couch."

Two psychiatrists were walking down a hall. One turned to the
other and said, "Good Morning!"
The other one thought, "I wonder what he meant by that?"

A middle-aged man was discussing his unique problem with
his psychiatrist. "You won't believe it, Doc. It's so trivial. I
know I really shouldn't get so worked up about it but I can't
help it, the thought seems to dominate every aspect of my
life."

"You've got me intrigued now," replies the shrink. "What is
it exactly that's bothering you?"

"Well I've collected all of the old Beatles singles. The
collection is my pride and joy. But I'm missing one single
and I just can't work out which one."

"I see," said the psychiatrist. "Well, this should be easy.
You've got A Hard Day's Night?"

"Yep!"

"She Loves You? I Want To Hold Your Hand? Twist and
Shout?"

"Uh-huh – I've got them all – except one."

The psychiatrist stroked his beard and thought for a
moment before saying: "What I think we have here is a
classic plea for Help!"

A woman went to her shrink because she was having severe problems with her sex life. The psychiatrist asked her many questions but did not seem to be getting a clear picture of her problems. Finally he asked, "Do you ever watch your husband's face while you are having sex?" "Well, yes, I actually did once."

"And how did your husband look?"

"Angry, very angry."

At this point the psychiatrist felt that he was really getting somewhere and he said, "Well that's very interesting, we must look into this further.

"Now tell me, you say that you have only seen your husband's face once during sex; that seems somewhat unusual. How did it occur that you saw his face that time?"

"He was looking through the window at us!"

A guy walks past a psychiatric hospital and hears a moaning voice "... 13 ... 13 ... 13 ..."

The man looks over to the hospital and sees a hole in the wall, he looks through the hole and gets poked in the eye. The moaning voice then groans "... 14 ... 14 ... 14 ..."

Depressed? Fatigued? Fed up at work? Just having a bad time all round? Why not try the seven steps of the latest stress management technique...

1. Picture yourself near a stream.

2. Birds are softly chirping in the cool mountain air.

3. No one but you knows your secret place.

4. You are in total seclusion from the hectic place called 'the world.'

5. The soothing sound of a gentle waterfall fills the air with a cascade of serenity.

6. The water is crystal clear.

7. You can easily make out the face of the person you're holding under the water.

You are feeling better already.

> *My psychiatrist told me he thought he'd worked out what my problem was: my inner child was adopted!*

My shrink told me I'm far too vain and I've got something called a 'narcissus complex'.
I think I need to take a good long look in the mirror.

> *I went on a train today and there were a load of manic depressive people running around screaming – turned out I was on the Bipolar Express.*

A newly qualified psychiatrist was questioning his patient. "Do you ever hear voices without being able to tell who is speaking or where the voices are coming from?" asked the psychiatrist.
"As a matter of fact, I do," said the patient.
The psychiatrist couldn't believe his luck. One of his first cases and he gets a classic case of schizophrenia. This was everything he dreamed of – no mild depression or mid-life crises, but a real mental illness. He was anxious to get more details. "So tell me," he asked. "How often do you hear these voices?"
"Oh, pretty much every time I answer the telephone." said his patient.

A guy goes to a psychiatrist. "Doc, I keep having these alternating recurring dreams. First I'm a tepee; then I'm a wigwam; then I'm a tepee; then I'm a wigwam. It's driving me crazy. What's wrong with me?" The doctor replies: "It's very simple. You're two tents."

A man walks into a psychiatrist's office wrapped in cling film with nothing underneath.
The psychiatrist says, "I can clearly see your nuts."

Question: How many psychiatrists does it take to change a light bulb?
Answer: That's an interesting question. What do you think?

A guy complains to his psychiatrist that he's been having strange dreams. "One night I dream I'm a Porsche, the next night I dream I'm a Trans Am – every night, I'm some kind of sports car. It's really starting to get to me." The psychiatrist responds, "Relax, you're just having an auto-body experience."

A man goes to see his psychiatrist. He says, "Doctor, I've been having suicidal tendencies. What should I do?"
The psychiatrist replies, "Pay your bill today."

Why is Saudi Arabia free of mental illness?

There are nomad people there.

Three women started boasting about their sons. "What a birthday I had last year!" exclaimed the first. "My son, that wonderful boy, threw me a big party in a fancy restaurant. He even paid for plane tickets for my friends."

"That's very nice, but listen to this," said the second. "Last winter, my son gave me an all-expenses-paid cruise to the Greek islands. First class."

"That's nothing!" interrupted the third. "For five years now, my son has been paying a psychiatrist £150 an hour, three times a week. And the whole time he talks about nothing but me."

I've just set fire to my psychiatrist's car. That'll teach him for saying I don't take criticism well.

A study conducted by Shrewsbury University's Department of Psychiatry has revealed that the kind of face a woman finds attractive on a man can differ depending on where she is in her menstrual cycle.

For example: If she is ovulating, she is attracted to men with rugged, masculine features.

However, if she is menstruating or menopausal, she tends to be more attracted to a man with scissors lodged in his temple and tape over his mouth while he is on fire.

No further studies are expected.

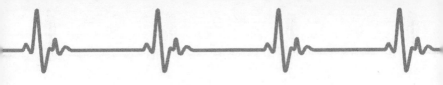

A psychiatrist sits behind his desk when he sees a man crawling on the floor.

"I guess you are a snake," he says.

The man does not reply and continues crawling.

"What are your worries, little snake?" the doc asks as the man crawls closer to him.

"What kind of snake are you?" he continues.

"For God's sake Doctor, knock it off," says the man. "I'm from the IT department and I am installing the Internet cable."

> *Did you hear about the constipated composer?*
> *He couldn't finish his last movement.*

The health minister is visiting a psychiatric ward. He asks the head of psychology, "How do you determine if a patient is cured?"

The psychologist explains: "We take them to the bathtub, which is filled with water, hand them a spoon and a cup and ask them to empty the bathtub."

"I see," says the health minister, "the cured person would choose the cup because it's bigger, and would empty the tub faster."

"Actually no," replies the psychologist, "a normal person would simply pull the plug."

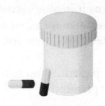

> *The psychology professor had just finished a lecture on mental health and was giving an oral test. Speaking specifically about manic depression, she asked, "How would you diagnose a patient who walks back and forth screaming at the top of his lungs one minute, then sits down weeping uncontrollably the next?" A young man in the rear raised his hand and answered, "A football manager?"*

A man goes to a psychologist and says, "Doc I got a real problem, I can't stop thinking about sex."

The psychologist says, "Well let's see what we can find out," and pulls out his ink blots. "What is this a picture of?" he asks.

The man turns the picture upside down then turns it around and states, "That's a man and a woman on a bed making love."

The psychologist says, "very interesting," and shows the next picture. "And what is this a picture of?"

The man looks and turns it in different directions and says, "That's a man and a woman on a bed making love."

The psychologists tries again with the third ink blot, and asks the same question, "What is this a picture of?"

The patient again turns it in all directions and replies, "That's a man and a woman on a bed making love."

The psychologist states, "Well, yes, you do seem to be obsessed with sex."

"Me!?" demands the patient. "You're the one who keeps showing me the dirty pictures!"

A general noticed one of his soldiers behaving oddly. The soldier would pick up any piece of paper he found, frown and say: "That's not it" and put it down again. This went on for some time, until the general arranged to have the soldier psychologically tested. The psychologist concluded that the soldier was deranged, and wrote out his discharge from the army.

The soldier picked it up, smiled and said: "That's it."

A doctor broke the bad news to a man, that his wife would have to be admitted to a psychiatric hospital. "I'm afraid her mind's completely gone," he said.

"Makes sense," mumbled the man. "She's been giving me a piece of it every day for the last 15 years."

"My shrink confirmed I've got an inferiority complex... but it's really not a very good one."

"My shrink diagnosed a serious problem with my tendency to extreme exhibitionism. Well, I'll show him..."

> *A guy went to a psychiatrist to get some help for his wife.*
> *"She's got a morbid fear of having her clothes stolen, doc", he told the psychiatrist.*
> *"Only two days ago I went home early and found she had hired a fellow to stay in the wardrobe and guard them."*

A patient said to a psychiatrist, "I keep wanting to cover myself in gold paint."
The psychiatrist said, "Sounds like you have a gilt complex."

Man: Doctor, my wife thinks she's a refrigerator!
Psychiatrist: Don't worry, it will pass.
Man: But Doctor, when she sleeps with her mouth open, the light keeps me awake!

"My therapist says that I've got a preoccupation with vengeance; we'll see about that..."

Last Trip to the Doctor's

Patient: Doctor, I think I swallowed a pillow.
Doctor: How do you feel?
Patient: A little down in the mouth.
Doctor: Have you ever had this before?
Patient: Yes.
Doctor: Well, you've got it again.

Frank is sitting in his living room when the doorbell rings. Upon answering the door, he finds a six foot tall cockroach that grabs him by the neck and beats him about the head and shoulders, then leaves.

The next night, the doorbell rings and it is the same 6 foot tall cockroach. He punches Frank in the abdomen and stalks off. The third night, the doorbell rings and it's the same six foot tall cockroach. This time he beats the snot out of poor Frank.

Frank staggers into the casualty department of his local hospital and collapses in triage. He looks at the nurse and says "Nurse, you gotta help me. I can't take any more of this!"

"Sorry," the nurse replies, "nothing we can do – there's a nasty bug going around."

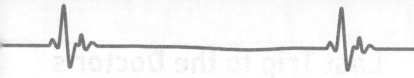

> *Just because a doctor has a name for your condition doesn't mean he knows what it is.*

After their 11th child a couple from Norfolk decide that's enough. The husband goes to his doctor and tells him that he wants the chop.

"Okay," says the doctor. "Go home, get a banger firework, light it, put it in a beer can, then hold the can up to your ear and count to ten."

The bumpkin replies, "I may not be the smartest man alive, but I don't see how putting a banger in a beer can next to my ear is going to help me." So, the man drives to London for a second opinion.

The London physician is just about to explain the procedure for a vasectomy when he notices from the case file that the man is from Norfolk. So instead the doc says, "Go home and get a banger, light it, place it in a beer can, hold to your ear and count to ten."

The bumpkin figures that both doctors can't be wrong, so he goes home, lights a banger and puts it in a beer can. He holds the can up to his ear and begins the countdown. "1, 2, 3, 4, 5...", at which point he pauses, places the beer can between his legs, and resumes counting on his other hand...

I went back to see my doctor today.
I said, "I applied the pile cream that you gave me this
morning and I got a very nasty reaction."
"Where exactly did you apply it?" he asked.
I said, "On the bus."

> *I went to the doctor's yesterday complaining of
> sore feet.*
>
> *He told me "Gout."*
>
> *I said "Come on, Doc. I've only just walked in!"*

Doctor: You seem to have jelly in one ear and custard in the other.
Patient: I have been feeling a trifle deaf.

"**Doctor, Doctor!** you've got to help me. I
think I'm a kleptomaniac."

*"Don't worry. I think there's
something you can take for that."*

I went to see the doctor today. He said, "I'm afraid you're suffering from a chronic case of denial."
I said, "I think I understand what you're saying. Basically I'm fine and there is a good chance I'll live forever?"

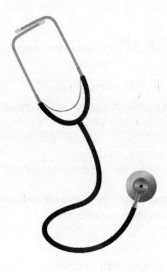

"Doctor, Doctor! I have a virus that makes my left hand constantly butter toast. How can I stop it spreading?"

"Doctor, Doctor! I keep thinking I'm a goat."

"How long have you had this feeling?"

"Ever since I was a kid."

> *The doctor had only examined her for a couple of minutes, but he pronounced, "I'd be prepared to hazard a guess that your daughter has got meningitis."*
> *I said "That's a little rash isn't it?"*

Doctor: What's wrong with your son?
Dad: He thinks he's a chicken.
Doctor: Really? How long has he thought this?
Dad: About three years.
Doctor: Three years! Why didn't you bring him in sooner?
Dad: We would have, but we needed the eggs.

I went to the doctors to see about my bad back. He asked me to walk across the room and back before telling me the real trouble was my posture. I had a feeling he might say that, but it was just a hunch.

158

A young woman went to see her doctor. "I'm really not feeling well, doctor," she explained. "From the moment I get up in the morning to when I go to bed at night I feel exhausted and I seem to catch every bug that's going around."

The doctor examined her thoroughly but could find no external symptoms. "I can't see anything wrong," he adds gently. "But I could sign you off work for a while."

"Oh that's ok." she replies. "I'm a fortune teller – it's not exactly physical work so I guess I'll struggle through."

A week later, the fortune teller is back at the surgery. "Sorry doctor," she says. "I know everyone will joke that I should have seen this coming, but I'm still feeling delicate and now I've come out in nasty blisters all over my body."

The doctor examined her again, still found nothing but took some tests and told her to return in a week.

A week later and the clairvoyant came back. "Still feeling weak?" asked the doc. She nodded. "Still blistered?"

"They've got worse," she said sadly.

"Any other symptoms developed?"

"Yes actually. Now I seem to have really bad breath all the time." she responded.

The doctor sighed and looked down at his notes. "Well, the tests don't tell me anything – I'm going to have to refer you to the experts." And with that he scribbled an admission note and sent her to the local hospital.

The fortune teller said goodbye and made her way to the hospital. On the bus she took out the note to see just what the doctor had written. "Please accept this patient for further examination," it read. "She appears to be a super-calloused fragile mystic plagued with halitosis."

Ron was terribly overweight, so his doctor put him on a diet.
"I want you to eat regularly for two days, then skip a day, and
repeat this procedure for 2 weeks. The next time I see you, you
will have lost at least five pounds."
When Ron returned, he shocked the doctor by losing nearly 20
pounds.
"Why, that's amazing!" the doctor said, "Did you follow my
instructions?"
Ron nodded. "I'll tell you, though, I thought I was going to drop
dead that third day."
"From hunger, you mean?"
"No, from skipping."

*A man went to his doctor complaining that
his get up and go had got up and gone. He no
longer seemed to be able to do all the things
around the house that he used to do. The doctor
performed a thorough examination and ran a
number of tests. A week later the guy returned
for the results.*
*"Now, Doc, give it to me straight. I can take it,"
he said. "Just tell me, in plain English, what is
wrong with me."*
*"Well, in plain English, absolutely nothing" his
doctor replied. "You're just plain lazy."*
*The patient thought for a second and then said.
"Okay, now give me the medical term so I can
tell my wife."*

Patient: Doctor, Doctor! I think I've turned into a pair
       of curtains.
Doctor: Pull yourself together, man!

A man developed a pain in his arm and decided to go to
the doctor. He arrived early and was checked in by the
receptionist who told him to give her a urine sample. "But
I'm not here for a check-up," the man replied. "I only have
a pain in my arm." "That's OK, sir. The doctor has a new
diagnostic machine to save time. Just leave a urine sample
and I will call you to come in when the test is complete."
The man was sceptical, and became irritated that the doctor
thought his machine was so good he didn't need to speak
with his patients. "So," he thought, "I'll teach him." He
asked to take the cup home and bring it in the next day. The
nurse agreed, and the man left.

When he got home, he explained everything to his family
and asked for their help. They agreed, and everyone
contributed a urine sample to the cup. The next day, before
he left, the man became cocky and added a little semen to
the cup. "This'll show him", thought the man. He then
delivered the specimen to the doctor's office.
Early the next day, the receptionist called the man to come
in "right away". After waiting only a few minutes, he was
called in to see the doctor. The doctor was leaning back
in his chair and giving the man the once over. The doctor
asked, with a wry smile on his face, "You think you're smart,
don't you?"
The man appeared surprised. "Well", the doctor said, "the
joke's on you. According to my analysis, your daughter's
pregnant, your wife has VD, your dog has the mange, and if
you don't stop beating off, you're never going to get rid of
that tennis elbow!"

Doctor: Have you taken my advice and slept with the
window open?
Patient: Yes.
Doctor: So your asthma disappeared completely?
Patient: No, but my ipad and my phone did.

**I went to the doctor the other day and said: "Doc, I find I'm
finishing crosswords too quickly, what can I do?"
The doctor replied: "Well, try not to get two down."**

My doctor entered the room.
"I'm not quite sure how to say this," he said, in a sombre tone.
"Oh my God," I sighed.
"Yes. It's one of those Latin words, really long with lots of 'y's,"
he snapped.

> *"I'm going to have to perform an emergency
> colostomy operation immediately."*
> the doctor told me.
> *"What's going to happen?" I asked.*
> *"It isn't pleasant. I'll have to remove part of your
> colon, and divert the rest of it to a hole in your
> side from which you will excrete into a bag for
> the rest of your life."*
> *"Is there an alternative?" I pleaded.*
> *"Yes, you can stop seeing my wife."*

I went to the doctors the other day to see if he could do anything about the sharp pain I was suffering in my back. He told me to take my shirt off and had a look. Then he said "Ahhh! You appear to have a huge key in your back, like some kind of clockwork toy."
I turned around and replied, "Are you winding me up?"

My wife went to the doctors the other day to see what might be causing her obesity problem. Turns out she has an over active knife and fork...

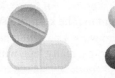

After having tried five operations and every pill available, the doctor was having a frank discussion with his patient. "There's really nothing more we can do to stop your terrible migraines, unless you'd consider trepanning."
"Great! I needed that news like I need a hole in the head!"

A hypochondriac patient broke down in front of his doctor.
"I'm sure I've got a liver disease, and I'm going to die from it."
"Ridiculous," said the doctor. "You'd never know if you had the disease or not. With that ailment there's no discomfort of any kind."
"Exactly," said the patient, "those are my exact symptoms."

Doctor: "I'm pretty sure you have an abnormal convex curvature of the thoracic vertebrae – but it's just a hunch!"

"Doctor, Doctor! , I keep thinking I'm a bottle of gin."

"I really think you could do with a little tonic."

An obese bloke goes to the doctor to see if he could help him lose weight. The doctor advised him to try a keep-fit DVD, But the guy said really wasn't going to work – he would never get round to doing the exercises.

"Well," suggested the doctor, "you really should try something that leaves you a little short of breath."

So the bloke took up smoking.

I went to the doctors. He said "Would you please lie on the couch."

I said, "Why's that Doc, do you think the problem is in my head?"

He replied "No. I just want to sweep the floor."

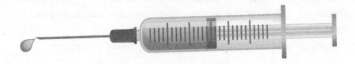

A woman rushes to see her doctor, looking incredibly worried and desperately stressed out. She blurts out: "Doctor, take a look at me. When I woke up this morning, I looked at myself in the mirror and saw my hair all wiry and frazzled, my skin was all wrinkled and pasty, my eyes were bloodshot and bugging out, and I had this corpse-like look on my face! What's on earth is wrong with me, Doctor!?"

The doctor looks her over for a couple of minutes, then calmly says: "Well, I can tell you that there's nothing wrong with your eyesight..."

A bloke goes in to the doctor and says, "Doc, I'm feeling kind of run down. Just don't have any energy, no get-up-and-go."

The doc gives him an exam, and finds nothing particularly noteworthy.

So, he starts asking about his lifestyle and diet. "What did you have for breakfast this morning?"

The man replied, "Snooker balls, just like every morning."

"Snooker balls! What kind?"

"Well, this morning, I had red ball, a purple ball, and a blue one. I also like the yellows, the oranges, and sometimes the black one, when I'm in the mood."

The doc smiles, and says, "I think I know what the problem is."

"What, doctor?"

"You're not eating enough greens."

Say 'Aaaaagh!'

Two doctors opened offices in a small town and put up a sign reading: 'Dr Smith and Dr Jones, Psychiatry and Proctology". The town council were not too happy with that sign, so they changed it to:

"Hysteria and Posteriors".

This was not acceptable either, so they changed the sign to:

"Schizoids and Haemorrhoids".

Still no go, so they tried:

"Manic-depressives and Anal-retentives."

This didn't get the nod either, so they tried:

"Minds and Behinds".

Nope. Nor:

"Analysis and Anal Cysts",

"Nuts and Butts",

"Freaks and Cheeks" or

"Loons and Moons"

So they finally settled on:

"Dr Smith and Dr Jones, Odds and Ends."

> *Two vampires walked into a bar and called for the bartender.*
> *"I'll have a glass of blood," said one.*
> *"I'll have a glass of plasma," said the other.*
> *"Okay," replied the bartender, "One glass of Blood and one Blood Lite coming up!"*

The owner of a garage was on the waiting list for a heart transplant. One day the phone rang and the lad in the office answered. It was the hospital with good news. "Hey Boss!" he yelled. "Your parts are in!"

A husband and wife were playing on the ninth green when she collapsed from a heart attack. "Please dear, I need help," she said. The husband ran off saying "I'll go get some help," A little while later he returned, picked up his club and began to line up his shot on the green.

His wife, on the ground, raised up her head and said, "I may be dying and you're putting?"

"Don't worry dear. I found a doctor on the second hole who said he'd come and help."

"The second hole??? When in the hell is he coming???"

"Hey! I told you not to worry," he said, practising stroking his putt. "Everyone's already agreed to let him play through."

Groves had been a butler for Lord Masterton's family all his life. But whilst attending his Lordship on a grouse shoot, Groves found himself on the wrong end of an accidental shot. He was rushed to hospital where they managed to save his life but unfortunately he had to have his arm amputated. When Groves came round after the operation, the surgeon was waiting with some good news and some bad news. "I'm afraid you've lost your right arm Groves, but the Masterton family felt so bad that they've kept your position as butler open and you will be able to return to work for them. The butler was immensely relieved and returned to service as soon as he could.

A month or so later, the surgeon was out shopping when he caught sight of a one-armed figure begging in a doorway. Back at his office he calls his Lordship to find out what happened.

"What happened? I thought you had agreed to keep Groves as your butler?"

"We did our best by the old chap," replied the Lord. "I did take him back. It was the least I could do. But in the end I had to let him go."

"The poor man. Why did you have to do that?"

"Well old bean, it's the same old problem with one-armed butlers: they can take it, but they can't dish it out.

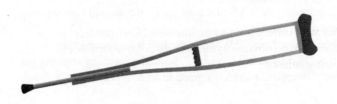

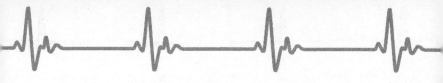

In a makeshift hospital tent in a bloody war zone, a soldier wakes up from surgery. "Doctor, doctor!" he yells. "There something wrong... I can't feel my legs!"
The doctor replies: "Ah Private Cole – that would be because we've had to amputate both your arms.

A 47-year-old woman is naked, jumping up and down on her bed laughing and singing. Her husband walks into the bedroom and sees her. He watches her a while then says, "You look ridiculous! What on earth do you think you're doing?"
She says, "I just got my check-up and my doctor says I have the breasts of an 18-year-old." She starts laughing and jumping up and down again.
He says, "Yeah, right. And what did he say about your 47-year old arse?"
She said, "Your name never came up."

> *Last night I was going to kill myself by swallowing a bottle of aspirins – but after taking the first two I felt much better.*

My wife suffers from a rare disease called Spendicitis. There are no obvious symptoms but it has a terrible effect on my balance.

"I've had it with my wife," said the one bloke to his mate.
"I'm filing for a divorce."
"I'm sorry to hear that," said his pal. "May I ask why?"
"I found her supply of birth control pills," said the first.
"Listen Joe, with all due respect to your religion, I can't
see you leaving your wife just because the Church says
it is a sin. Things are changing in the world. There are
many Catholics who deem it perfectly acceptable to use
contraceptives. You need to get with the times, mate."
"It ain't just that." argued Joe. "I had a vasectomy over five
years ago."

During the BSE scare a couple went to dinner at an exclusive
restaurant in London.
The man ordered a fillet steak, prepared rare.
The waiter asks politely, "Ok, but what about the mad cow, Sir?"
"Oh don't worry," answers the man, "she'll order for herself ..."

An African chief was feeling very sick, so he summoned
the witch doctor to his hut. After a brief examination, the
medicine man cut off a thong of antelope hide from his belt
and gave it to the chief, instructing him to bite off, chew,
and swallow one inch of leather every day. After one month,
the witch doctor returned, and asked how the chief was
feeling. The chief answered, "The thong is ended, but the
malady lingers on."

"Hello is that 555555?"
"Yes."
"Can you call an ambulance for me? I've glued my finger to the
phone!"

> *What do you call a woman driving an Ambulance? ... Nina!*

An ambulance with its siren blaring passed by my brother-in-law's house. After they passed the house, they noticed a figure running as fast as he could behind the ambulance. Concerned, the ambulance driver stopped the ambulance. His colleague got out the van and asked the brother-in-law if he was ok. After a minute or two, when he had his breath back, the idiot looked up and asked, "Err, do you have any ninety-nines?"

Paddy rings an ambulance for his mate Mick. "Come quick, my mate Mick is hurt and needs help fast."

The operator tells Paddy to calm down and asks the location of the victim. "He's at 104 Eucalyptus Boulevard." says Paddy.

"Can you spell that please," asks the operator. The line goes quiet and the operator says "Hello Sir. Are you still there?"

Minutes pass and the operator is about to give up when Paddy comes back on the line. "Right, I've just dragged him to 2 Oak Road."

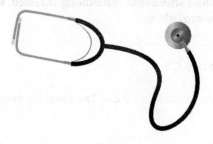

The emergency services had an interesting call last week from the local furniture shop. A guy had fallen into the automatic upholstering machine. It was ok, though. The hospital said he's fully recovered.

A 92-year-old woman had a full cardiac arrest at home and was rushed to the hospital. After 30 minutes of unsuccessful resuscitation attempts the old lady was pronounced dead. The doctor went to tell the lady's 78-year old daughter that her mother didn't make it. "Didn't make it? That's impossible. Where could they be? She left in the ambulance forty-five minutes ago!"

I gave the ambulance men the wrong blood type for my ex – now she knows what rejection feels like!

A General Practitioner is a doctor who keeps knowing less and less about more and more areas until he knows nothing about everything. A specialist on the other hand, knows more and more about less and less until he knows everything about nothing.

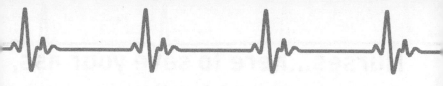

Three paramedics were boasting about improvements in their respective ambulance team's response times.

"Since we installed our new satellite navigation system," bragged the first one, "we cut our emergency response time by ten percent."

The other paramedics nodded in approval. "Not bad," the second paramedic commented. "But by using a computer model of traffic patterns, we've cut our average response time by 20 percent."

Again, the other team members gave their congratulations, until the third paramedic said, "That's nothing! Since our ambulance driver passed his law exam, we've cut our emergency response time in half!"

As the ambulance pulls up to the scene of a car crash, the driver looks across at the pink, upturned Nova. He fetches his medical kit and races across to the vehicle, crouching to examine the blonde girl at the wheel of the battered car. As he studies the red smears on the upholstery, he asks, "Can you tell me where you're bleeding from?"

"Essex," she replies.

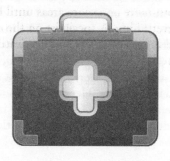

Nurses...here to save your ass, not kiss it!

Did you hear about the nurse who swallowed a razor blade? She gave herself a tonsillectomy, an appendectomy, a hysterectomy, and circumcised three of the doctors on her shift.

Did you hear about the nurse who died and went straight to hell? It took her two weeks to realize that she wasn't at work anymore!

How many triage nurses does it take to change a light bulb? One, but the bulb will have to spend four hours in the waiting room.

A nurse delivered a lunch tray to her patient, Mr Jones, and also gave him a urine specimen utensil, adding that when he was able, he should put a specimen in the glass and she'd pick it up when she came back to get the tray. The patient, seeing some apple juice on the tray and without thinking, poured some into the specimen glass. The nurse came back and picked up the specimen, held it up to the light and said, "Mr Jones, this doesn't looks good. The colour doesn't seem quite right. Are you feeling okay?" Mr Jones reached out his hand for the glass and said, "Here, let me look." Realizing what had happened, he said, "Okay, I'll run it through again." To the nurse's amazement he raised the glass and downed it in one gulp!

Two staff nurses and a senior nurse at the hospital were taking a lunch break in the break room. Suddenly in walks a lady dressed in brightly-coloured silk scarves. "I am 'Gilda the Great'," stated the lady. "I am so grateful for the way you have taken care of my aunt that I will now grant you a wish each!" With a wave of her hand and a puff of smoke, the room was filled with flowers, fruit and bottles of drink, proving to the astonished onlookers that she did have the power to grant wishes.

The nurses quickly argued among themselves as to which one would ask for the first wish. Speaking up, a staff nurse wished first. "I wish I were on a tropical island beach, with beautiful men feeding me fruit and tending to my every need." With a puff of smoke, the nurse was gone.

The other staff nurse went next." I wish I were rich and retired and spending my days in my own warm cabin at a ski resort with well-groomed men feeding me cocoa and doughnuts." With a puff of smoke, she too was gone.

"Now, what is the last wish?" asked the lady.

The Senior nurse then said," I want those two back in the ward by the end of the lunch break."

Three doctors are in the hallway complaining about one of the nurses.

"She's out of control!" the first doctor says. "She does everything backwards. Just last week I told her to give a man two milligrams of morphine every ten hours. She gave him 10 milligrams every two hours, he almost died!"

"That's nothing," said the second doctor, "earlier this week I told her to give a man an enema every 24 hours, she tried to give him 24 enemas in one hour!"

All of a sudden they heard a blood curdling scream from down the hallway. "Oh my God!" cried the third. "I just realized that I told her to prick Mr. Smith's boil!"

A man is lying in bed in hospital with an oxygen mask over his mouth. A young trainee nurse arrives to sponge his face and hands.

"Nurse, he mumbles from behind the mask, "are my testicles black?"

Embarrassed the young nurse replies, "I really don't know, I'm only here to wash your face and hands."

He struggles again to ask, "Nurse, are my testicles black?"

Once again the nurse replies, "I wouldn't know. I'm just to give you a quick wash."

The senior nurse is passing and sees the man getting a little upset so marches over to inquire what was wrong.

"Nurse," he mumbles, "are my testicles black?"

Having seen much worse, the senior nurse doesn't care. She pulls back the bedclothes, whips down his pyjama trousers, moves his dick out of the way, gives them a quick once over, pulls up the pyjamas, replaces the bedclothes and announces, "Nothing wrong with them!!!"

At this the man pulled off his oxygen mask and asks again, "I was only asking, are my test results back?"

You know you're a nurse if...

🚑 You've been telling stories in a restaurant and had someone at another table throw up.

🚑 You own at least three pens with the names of prescription medications on them.

🚑 You're at the grocery checkout and you are summing up their veins.

- You wash your hands before going to the bathroom, as well as after.

- You no longer have a gag reflex.

- You consider a tongue depressor an eating utensil.

- You've been exposed to so many X-rays that youconsider it a form of birth control.

- You've ever bet on someone's blood alcohol level.

- You believe you have patients who are demonically possessed.

- You start to worry if your patient hasn't urinated in a few hours, but you've gone almost the entire shift without making it to the loo.

- You hear the beeping from a truck reversing, you jump up to see whose alarm is going off.

- You ask your father-in-law what colour his stool is and when is the last time he moved his bowels.

- You unconsciously take your husband's or wife's pulse when you hold his/her hand.

- You can empty a bedpan while eating a egg mayonnaise sandwich.

A big-shot business man was booked into a private ward in the hospital. He was a complete pain in the arse, bossed the nurses around like he owned them. None of the hospital staff wanted to have anything to do with him.

The senior nurse was the only one who could stand up to him. She walked into his room and announced, "I have to take your temperature."

After complaining for several minutes, he finally settled down, crossed his arms and opened his mouth.

"No, I'm sorry, the nurse stated, "but for this reading, I can't use an oral thermometer."

This started another round of complaining, but eventually he rolled over and bared his behind.

After feeling the nurse insert the thermometer, he heard her announce, "I have to get something. Now you stay just like that until I get back!"

She left the door to his room open on her way out. He curses under his breath as he heard people walking past his door, laughing. After almost an hour, the man's doctor came into the room.

"What's going on here?" asked the doctor.

Angrily, the man answered, "What's the matter, Doc? Haven't you ever seen someone having their temperature taken before?"

After a pause, the doctor replied, "Yes, but never with a daffodil!"

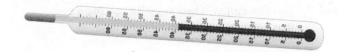

I told my GP I couldn't afford the time to go to hospital for an operation. He was pretty decent about it – he touched up my x-rays.

The hospital had a Nurse called 'The Appendix'.
All the surgeons in the hospital had taken her out.

Heard about the nurse who was marrying the X-ray specialist? Everyone wondered what it was he saw in her.

What did the nurse say when she found a rectal
thermometer in her pocket?
"Some asshole has my pen!"

> *A new nurse listened while the doctor was*
> *yelling, "Typhoid! Tetanus! Measles!"*
> *The new nurse asked another nurse, "Why is he*
> *doing that?"*
> *The other nurse replied, "Oh, he just likes to*
> *call the shots around here."*

It was a nurse's first day and her manager was ascertaining to what level she had been trained. "Now nurse," asked the manager. "Imagine a man's been brought in after an accident and he's vomiting, distressed and bleeding badly. Could you tell me what would be the first thing that you would do?"
The nurse thought for a second and replied: "Faint."

A senior nurse walks into a hospital waiting room and is greeted with an unmistakable odour. "OK," she shouts. "Who messed in their pants?" No one answers. Determined to get to the bottom of the stench, she walks around to each patient. Finally she finds the culprit, an old drunk in the corner. "Hey," she says. "How come you didn't answer when I asked who messed in their pants?"
"Oh," replies the drunk. "I thought you meant today."

The young nurse was nervous about giving vaccinations but gave it her best shot.

Jerry is recovering from an operation when a nurse asks him how he is feeling.
"I'm OK but I didn't like the four-letter-word the doctor used in surgery," he answered.
"What did he say," asked the nurse.
"OOPS!"

Hear about the surgery nurse who was disciplined for being absent without gauze?

The nurse had shown the man into a cubicle but he was clearly not happy.

"OK sir," she said. "What's the problem here?"

"Well nurse," he began. "Maybe I should go – you'll only laugh at me."

"I'm a professional," she replies. "In over twenty years, I've never yet laughed at a patient."

"Okay then," said the patient, and he proceeded to drop his trousers, revealing the smallest male part the nurse had ever seen. In length and width, it was almost identical to an AAA battery.

Unable to control herself, the nurse tried to stop a giggle, but it just came out. Feeling very bad that she had laughed at the tiny member, she composed herself as well as she could.

"I am so sorry," she said, "I don't know what came over me. On my honour as a nurse, I promise that won't happen again. Now, tell me, what seems to be the problem?"

"It's my penis," Bob replied. "It's terribly swollen."

Doctor: Nurse, how is that little girl doing who swallowed those pound coins last night?

Nurse: There's no change yet.

Guess who I bumped into in the optician's...? EVERYBODY!

Optician: Have your eyes been checked before?

Startled patient: No. They've always both been blue!

Yesterday I went to the opticians, walked up to the counter and said to the girl on the desk, "I think my eyes are going." Quick as a flash she said, "They've gone mate – this is Burger King."

Did you hear the one about the optician who fell into the lens grinder? He made a spectacle of himself.

In the opticians one of the sales staff was trying to convince a customer that she needed a stronger prescription.
"It's ok. I'm fine with what I have," insisted the customer.
"You think so?" he challenged, "well, what does it say on the shop window across the street?"
As quick as anything she replied "50% off everything."
"That's incredible," admitted the sales assistant. "I take it back. Your vision is perfect."
"Not really," confessed the customer. "But I never miss a sale!"

Dave and Paul are playing golf together, they usually have a close match but suddenly Dave seems so much better. All his drives head straight for the pin and he sinks every putt first time. He ends up winning by 14 strokes.

So Paul asks Dave how come his game got so good. "It's these new super bifocals my optician got me," his mate tells him. "I look out the top of the glasses when I am driving and the pin looks as if it's only 50 yards away. Then when I get on the green I look out the bottom half and the hole looks the size of a dustbin lid. I never realised how it could improve my game."

A few weeks later they meet up at the clubhouse bar. Dave has now got himself some new super bifocals. He buys a round then goes to the toilet. But when he comes out his trousers are absolutely drenched with pee.

"Dave, what on earth happened?" asks Paul.

"It's these new glasses," his friend replies. "When I looked down I could see two instead of one. Well, I guessed the big one was mine, so I put the other one away..."

"Hmm..." said the optician at the man's check up. "I prescribed those glasses because you were seeing fuzzy spots in front of your eyes. Have they helped at all?" "Oh yes," replied the patient. "The spots are much clearer now."

A man goes to the opticians. "I keep seeing spots in front of my eyes," says the man. "Have you ever seen a doctor?" asks the optician. "No, replies the man, just spots."

Clive had lived a long life, which was drawing to its end. As his family surrounded him on his deathbed, he asked to see his optician.

"An optician?" they asked. "Why in the world do you want to see your optician?"

"Just get him for me."

So they get the eye-doctor, who, on seeing Clive about to depart this life, asked, "Clive, it pains me to see you like this. What can I possibly do for you?"

Clive opened his eyes slightly and said, "Before I go, there's one thing I have to know. Which one was clearer – A or B?"

A Czech man went to the opticians to have his eyes tested. The optician pointed to a chart on the wall that displayed the letters F T W K P W X S C Z Y and asked if he could read it. "Can I read it?" the Czech man replied "He was my next door neighbour!"

A man goes to the opticians and says "Can you help me? I'm suffering from double vision."

"Take a seat please," says the optician.

"Which one?" the man replies.

Die? That's The Last Thing I'll Do!

A doctor was just starting out on his own, when he found that he had too much work to do. Now this man was brilliant, and had particularly good people skills. Once he got a patient, they just would not see anyone else.

It seems that this man had been reading recently about the advances in cloning, and decided to have a clone made of himself to do his work.

For years it worked perfectly. His clone took care of all his patients and he got to relax. However, as happens with clones, it wasn't quite perfect. The clone had some personality disorders. It would insult patients using the foulest of language. It got so bad that business was suffering. The doctor decided that he just had to get rid of the clone or risk losing his business.

So he took his clone for walk along the cliff and when he had the opportune moment he pushed the clone over to his death.

The doctor again began seeing his old patients and things were going exceptionally well, until the clone was washed up on the shore. The police were baffled. The real doctor was obviously alive, and the dead body was a clone – they didn't know just what to charge the doctor with. After much deliberation, they decided to charge him with... Making an obscene clone fall.

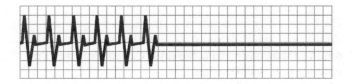

Bert came home from the doctor looking very worried.

His wife said, "What's the problem?"

He said, "The doctor told me I have to take a pill every day for the rest of my life."

She said, "So what? Lots of people have to take a pill every day their whole lives."

He said, "I know, but he only prescribed me four pills!"

A man goes to the doctors and asks why he's been feeling ill. The doctor examines him and replies "I'm sorry to tell you, you've got the disease known as Yellow 24." "What's that?" the man asks. "It means your internal organs have started turning yellow - you've got 24 hours to live."

The man goes home and tells his wife the bad news. His wife says "Well, will you come to bingo with me tonight then? Otherwise you'll never be able to."

The man agrees so he and his wife go to the bingo. He finds that he's won the one-line and £10. He begins to think this isn't such a bad day after all. Twenty minutes later, he's won the full house and £150. He enters the lucky draw, worth £500, and wins that too. The bingo caller calls him up on stage.

He says "I don't believe it, mate. You've won three competitions and a total of £660 in one night. You must be the luckiest man on earth!"

The man says "Well, no, I'm not. I found out today that I've got Yellow 24."

The bingo caller looks down at the piece of paper he's holding and starts clapping. "I don't believe it; he's only gone and won the raffle as well!"

A man goes to the doctor and he finds out that he is very ill and only has a few weeks to live. He can't believe it and pleads with the doctor, "This is a disaster Doc. There must be something you can do?"

The doctor says that unfortunately it is too late for treatment. He needs to face facts and he should concentrate on getting his affairs in order.

"There must be something!" the man says. "What about radiation, Chemotherapy... I'm a tough guy!"

The doctor again says that there is nothing they can do for him and he should concentrate on using the time he has left wisely.

The man, however, is beside himself and will not give up. "Doc, please. What about experimental treatments? I'm not leaving until you give me something!"

At this point the doctor finally says, "OK, if I were you I'd take my wife up to the wine country and go to one of those spas they have. Get yourself a good a mud bath."

Now the guy senses there is possibly a way out after all. "A mud bath?" he says. "OK, I'll try anything but why Doc? How come if radiation won't work and chemo won't work, a mud bath is somehow going to heal me?"

"Ah, replies the Doctor, "it isn't going to heal you – but it will get you used to dirt."

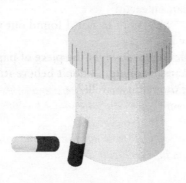

Lawyer: Before you signed the death certificate, had you taken the pulse?
Pathologist: No.
Lawyer: Did you listen to the heart?
Pathologist: No.
Lawyer: Did you check for breathing?
Pathologist: No.
Lawyer: So, when you signed the death certificate you weren't actually sure he was dead, were you?
Pathologist: Well, let me put it this way. The man's brain was sitting in a jar on my desk. But I guess it's possible he could be out there practising law somewhere.

A woman goes into the local newspaper office to see that the obituary for her recently deceased husband is published. After the editor informs her that the fee for the obituary is 50p a word, she pauses, reflects and then says, "Well, then, let it just read 'Arnold Green died'." Amazed at the woman's tight-fistedness, the editor explains that there is a 7-word minimum for all obituaries. The woman pauses again, counts on her fingers and replies, "In that case, 'Arnold Green died: 2006 Volkswagen for sale'."

John was on his deathbed and gasped pitifully.
"Give me one last request, dear," he said.
"Of course, John," his wife said softly.
"Six months after I die," he said, "I want you to marry Bob."
"But I thought you hated Bob," she said.
With his last breath John said, "I do!"

> *I had a mate who was suicidal.*
> *He was really depressed, told me I had to help*
> *him die – it was his only wish. So I pushed him*
> *in front of a steam train.*
> *He was chuffed to bits.*

When the husband finally died his wife put the usual death notice in the paper, but added that he died of gonorrhoea. No sooner were the papers delivered when a friend of the family phoned and complained bitterly, "You know very well that he died of diarrhoea, not gonorrhoea."

The widow replied, "I nursed him night and day so of course I know he died of diarrhoea, but I thought it would be better for posterity to remember him as a great lover rather than the big shit he always was."

A mortician was working late one night. It was his job to examine the dead bodies before they were sent off to be buried or cremated. As he examined the body of Mr Lovett, who was about to be cremated, he made an amazing discovery. Lovett had the longest private part he had ever seen!

"I'm sorry, Mr. Lovett," said the mortician to the dead man, "but I can't send you off to be cremated with a tremendously huge private part like this. It has to be saved for posterity."

With that, the coroner used his tools to remove the dead man's unit. He stuffed his prize into a briefcase and took it home. The first person he showed it to was his wife.

"I have something to show you that you won't believe," he said, and opened up his briefcase.

"Oh my God!" the wife screamed, "Lovett is dead!"

A bloke's wife goes missing while diving off the West Australian coast. He reports the incident, searches fruitlessly and spends a terrible night wondering what could have happened to her.

Next morning there's a knock at the door and he is confronted by a couple of policemen, the old Sergeant and a younger Constable. The Sergeant says, "Mate, we have some news for you. Unfortunately some really bad news, but some good news, and maybe some more good news."

"Well," says the bloke, "I guess I'd better have the bad news first."

The Sergeant says, "I'm really sorry mate, but your wife is dead. Young Bill here found her lying at about five fathoms deep in a little dip in the reef. He got a line around her and we pulled her up, but I'm afraid to say she was dead."

The bloke is naturally pretty distressed to hear of this he sits himself down and has a little cry. But after a few minutes he pulls himself together and asks, "Hey, didn't you say there was some good news – what's that about, fellas?"

The Sarge says, "Well, when we pulled your wife up, there were quite a few really good sized crays and a swag of nice crabs attached to her, so we've brought you your share."

He hands the bloke a string bag with a couple of nice crayfish and four or five crabs in it.

"Geez thanks. They're bloody beauties. I guess it's an ill wind and all that... So what's the other possible good news?"

"Well," the Sarge says, "if you fancy a quick trip, me and young Bill here get off duty at around 11 o'clock and we're gonna drive over there and pull her up again...!"

The Grim Reaper came for me last night, and I beat him off with a vacuum cleaner.
Talk about Dyson with death.

Mary O'Leary goes up to Father O'Hannigan after his Sunday morning service. She's in a terrible state, crying and hollering.

He says, "So what's bothering you, Mary my dear?"

She says, "Oh, Father, I've got terrible news. My husband passed away last night."

The priest says, "Oh, Mary, that's terrible. Tell me, Mary, did he have any last requests?"

She says, "That he did, Father."

The priest says, "What did he ask, Mary?"

She says, "He said, 'Please Mary, put down that damn gun...'"

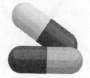

A dying man smells his favourite scones cooking downstairs. It takes all the strength he has left but he gets up from the bed and crawls down the stairs. He sees the scones cooling on the counter and staggers over to them. As he reaches for one, his wife's hand reaches out, smacks his and she yells: "No, you can't have those! They're for the funeral!"

A man phoned his heart surgeon to schedule an appointment for an immediate surgery.
"I'm sorry," the receptionist answered, "we don't have anything available for the next three weeks."
"But I could die by then!" he argues.
The receptionist however, was not to be swayed: "No problem, if that happens just give us a call to cancel the appointment."

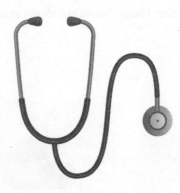